MY BOY

First Published in the UK 2012 by Mirador Publishing

First edition: 2012

A copy of this work is available through the British Library.

ISBN: 978-1-908200-74-7

Mirador Publishing
Mirador
Wearne Lane
Langport
Somerset
TA10 9HB

Acknowledgements:

Love and thanks to the wonderful staff at St Richard's Hospice, Worcester, England and all those involved in the palliative care programmes.

To my good friends Dai Gealy, Lorretta McCloughlin, whose kindness and encouragement have made a great difference.

Cover by Genesiscreatives.com

CHAPTER ONE

I suppose I let him slip away from me when he was alive. I loved him of course but took for granted that my life was to be nurtured first, after all we'd given him a good education and a good home.

But slip away he did, to a world I could not imagine. It was imperceptible; he drifted away from me and my new wife. His lifestyle was foreign to me, he was an amiable nuisance. I kept a lazy eye on him, fretting more about my social niceties than what was before my very eyes.

Over the years we met, after a fifty mile tedious drive we'd often spend forty minutes or less together and he'd be off, usually with a few quid from his Dad. He pleaded poverty and an endless tale of misfortune. I believed him because I chose to, because I could not bear to admit he was a drug addict.

With this truth staring me in the face, I dismissed everything else; his way of life, his partner, his kids. I wanted to be his father but without the unbearable inconvenience of his way of living. I loved him and expressed that love in a constant stream of admonishment about pulling himself together and getting a grip – of what I was never prepared to define!

And so his life almost passed me by, he lay in my head each day, a worry – a frustration and a care. Yes I loved him, but I was so bad at it. I wonder every day, if he knew? I hope so. I even believe so, not to comfort myself, but because from his side of his life I learned that he was a good boy, a man who loved his kids better than I had mine. He understood his addiction and lived with it, and even enjoyed much of his life style which was wild, exciting and sometimes full of fun. He knew too, how dark it could get, how the addiction could squeeze his being with pain beyond my understanding.

So when I came home one day and my daughter told me he was in hospital, I was not altogether surprised – he'd not been looking good for some time. During our infrequent and short meetings he'd looked gaunt and unwell. I was assured he was fine. This time though he was in hospital with pleurisy; worrying certainly, but before I knew he was out of hospital again, and from the distance I thought not too much of it. He was apparently fine - wasn't that good to know!

Then the dreadful day, the inevitable, the day that in my heart I knew was coming, the word was cancer, he was back in hospital and for once I did not prevaricate I went to be with him. I did not go to visit, I went to be with him and within a split second on that awful day I knew my son was dying.

The vigil started with the uncertainty of an unfamiliar institution, the medical assessment ward where he lay.

They talk of methadone and addiction and for the first time we look each other in the eye, acknowledge each other and I say nothing. His sister, my lovely daughter leads me through the emotions of these long days. I, determined through her strength, that I will be with him through the difficult steps ahead, when hope will be taken away, when he walks through the valley of darkness to an inevitably rough and painful end.

Being in hospital is not what anyone wants, especially a boy, my boy, whose life had been a constant slavery to addiction for how many years? I could only guess. I begin to imagine how he'd spent day after day being ruled by his habit, pretending to have to be somewhere else to get his fix. His shame, his fear, that we would discover his way of life; his consequent inability to engage with us. Worst of all, we conspire with him; we turn away, or look at him with our collective blind eye.

But now he is captive he can't slip away, he can go to the entrance of the Hospital and join that hapless group of tobacco addicts as they sit gasping at their cigarettes, most knowing that they are killing themselves. I try not to, but I come to loathe the collection of smokers, their lemming like behaviour reminding me that my boy is just like them.

Inside the hospital itself the overwhelming feeling is that no one on the staff gives a damn about individuals, the possible exception being the porters, who are a jolly lot, mainly from Eastern Europe. The porters are unfailingly cheerful and I came to know a number by their first names. As I trail along behind them as we sweep my boy to his many nameless appointments, they keep up a chatter that is both kind and amusing. There is not much amusement anywhere else. I seldom see the same nurse more than twice and that is a rarity. None of them come to my boy to comfort him, nor to offer a smile. It is always a duty roster, to deliver pills or fill in a chart. They may be nurses but they aren't carers. I hold the guilty feeling that their feeling toward my boy is just like mine toward the smokers at the front door.

The wards are bewildering and my boy is moved from an observation ward which is overcrowded and has both male and female patients, to another medical ward where there were a small number of males; all very ill. We watch his neighbours die off, he seems stoic; he still believes that he is made of sterner stuff.

Each of the wards has junior doctors who seem to spend most of the days behind the office desk. When I enquire about my son, they inevitably avoid engagement. Sometimes I corner them, and still they evade any helpful conversation, as if I am a half wit who wouldn't understand. These junior doctors all disappear at five o'clock sharp and are never to be seen at weekends – all to do with a European directive I am told. Patients sadly continued to suffer and call for pain killers which have to be signed off by a doctor in the evenings and at weekends. There is no directive for their suffering.

There are endless waits and walks down unending corridors, to canteen and restaurants where he eats prodigious amounts of cake and coffee, where we talk for hours about nothing. We don't speculate about his prognosis, I avoid the subject; he occasionally mentions a test that he must undergo. We are both by and large ignored by the nursing staff who look at him as a lost cause. There is a resigned view when he asked for pain killers, an unsaid "tut tut," 'druggies' must wait their turn for morphine or whatever he needs. There are problems injecting him because his veins were no longer serviceable, so try as they may, it is impossible to intravenously feed any treatment into him. A very experienced ward nurse tries with great patience and gentleness to get a line into him, and ten minutes later a disinterested nurse accidentally pulls out the drip. He is never to have another and the consequences will be dire.

The Hospital has little sympathy for a smoking junkie who's brought these trials on himself. Kindness is fleeting, impatience frequent and disdain constant. He knows it and sees it and yet he does not respond with anger. I am angry, part of me angry with him, part of me angry with them. Can't they find some generosity of spirit to make him feel he was worth something? His physical state is appalling, ulcerated leg, skeletal emaciation, he looks awful, he looks a wreck who nobody would want to love. But he was loved by his sister and his kids and his mum and dad, though his kids and mother see only illness, not imminent death.

Discoveries, oh what discoveries? I piece together the history, of the earlier messages of months before. When the boy was briefly in hospital earlier, some months before, it transpired because he was interned over a weekend when there were no doctors on duty and so no diagnosis of his medical condition, or his addiction, he discharged himself to get a fix, and in that fleeting moment had probably sacrificed any hope of survival.

My wife, comes with me and meets the first drug addict of her life – my son. He is strangely relaxed and at ease, partly because my wife is beautiful and radiates kindness. These two people who I love with all my heart accept each other without a thought.

Test followed test, and he hangs on believing that this will end with healing. He whispers to me that the technicians had mentioned abscess in the lung, hope then, I encourage him to believe in the impossible.

I know with a certainty that this is not to be. And then the fateful day when all would be revealed, the doctors will pronounce the way ahead. What time? When? Two o'clock, three o'clock, four o'clock – Christ save us! Five o'clock.

"Can't operate, can't cure..." I hear the words, I knew them before they were uttered, I want to bite my tongue out, I want to stop the words being said. And then the Doctor's gone - we hug. He asks, "what does it mean?" We hug again, I must not cry. I hold him- a bag of terrible bones, he flinches because my hug hurts him. The cancer is in his bones, in his spine, it's everywhere, it's obscene, and it's killing my son, now, right now – here in my arms, and I must not cry.

"You'll manage I tell him, it's part of the human spirit, and I'll be here all the way." We hug again. How long? How Long? How Long? I promise he will never know. We hug again, and lo and behold his pal turns up to visit. My son smiles he's glad to see his pal.

I meet a hospital sister who is a specialist in these matters – matters of the terminally ill, the condemned. Her uniform was smart, her smile reassuring. There was to be some more treatment at another hospital where my boy will be given radiotherapy and that will bring temporary comfort. And then as casually as if discussing the weather, it was made clear that my son was to be discharged into my care. The cancer radiology centre appointment is at another hospital a further fifty long miles away from my home and they will receive us on the morrow.

I go to tell his mother, it will be hard, this is a very hard day. She is a sweet woman, who has lived in the same house as my son for eight years. He has come and gone silently resisting all her efforts to feed him, and to look after him, she has scrimped and saved to keep him and he has no doubt squeezed money from her just as he did from me. She, I know, loved him like me but has lived through everyday, watching, fretting, afraid, with much more pain. Like me, she had chosen not to see the obvious nature of his drug addiction, or else to deny it. There is a part of me that was angry with her. But who am I to criticise?

I knock on her door, she lets me in, I peck her on the cheek, she sits. There is no easy way of telling a mother her son is to die. I repeat the doctor's words with little pre-amble except, "Look the news is not good, they can't operate and they can't cure." She looks at me and I watch the barb strike home. She wails, a sound of an agonised soul, and I rush to her side and hold her, and stroke her hair, something I have not done for twenty five years. She sobs; "My baby, my baby.." For the first time I have a glimpse of the meaning of motherhood. Flesh of her flesh, part of her is dying – her agony is more profound than I can imagine. We weep together, I release my hold, she sits again.

"How long?"

"I don't know but not very long," I say. "They say not more than a year, but who knows and who am I to guess, but our poor boy has less than that. How much less I have no idea."

We talk, he must come home, yes, he must come home. We must do our best. We talk of managing his homecoming, she is already planning to bring his bed downstairs. Eventually I leave, for once I feel for her and understand that whatever went before, no mother could have loved him more. My guilt stirred uncomfortably on the journey home, my next job is to tell my daughter.

I return to the hospital and collect my son, I take him home to his mum's, where already a bed had been brought downstairs. I pile him into my car with a huge collection of bottles and boxes of drugs, we make the journey to his mother's house, his home these last eight years, in silence. He is glad to leave the Hospital, he smiles and looks forward to impossible dreams, of comfort and fun and liberty.

He lights a cigarette, I curse and shout at him – it's killing him – so what?

CHAPTER TWO

I leave him in his mother's care. I feel unsure, to stay or go. There is my daughter, his daughter and his mother – I feel unnecessary, a super numery, I have nothing to offer. These girls of three generations all muck in – he is submerged in love.

I leave. He seems glad to be home. In the car I worry that he needs a bath and a shave. I worry about his dignity – or is it my dignity? I am still lousy as a father. I drive the long disconsolate journey to my home and my lovely wife who will be my safe harbour. I weep as I drive staggering into traffic jams, marooned and sorry, sorry for me and disconsolate for my boy. A motorway was never so lonely at rush hour.

I phone my daughter and we cry some more, illegally phoning – maybe crying is illegal too. His mum tells me he's settling. The journey home is long, I shall know this journey well as the days tick by, each day closer to the next and to the last.

The next day I drive to him and we go to the radiotherapy clinic some fifty miles further distant. He's had a mixed night and he packs his drugs and pain killers to last the journey. He complains that he doesn't have enough and that the pain is relentless. He is very restless, I try and talk about anything to keep him engaged, he swigs his Oramorph and squirms in his seat. I find I have to be careful what I say. I cannot talk of the future we both know there's not much of that.

We arrive in the county town and find the Hospital and the radiology centre; parking is chaotic, I drop him off at the entrance and set out to find a parking spot. It is a cold and rainy day, the hospital exterior is a rambling hotch-potch of dull low buildings. I rush back to his side and we weave our way through a myriad of corridors toward the radiotherapy centre. He finds it hard to walk, so we stop and I go and find a wheelchair. We find the allotted space and wait, he is in great pain; he is losing it. He is dancing on the balls of his feet and clutching his chest in his spindly arms. He swears and curses out loud, other patients look alarmed. I admonish him, "Hang on, hold on," I am crying and the tears are rolling down my face, I hug him and he pushes me away because to hug is to hurt. I am desperate, desperate in my way as he is in his, we are utterly lost, we need someone, anyone who can help us. I squeeze my eyes and pray, I dare any of the astonished patients to say anything, I will kill them- I will!

Then we are called to a small examination room where my shivering, dancing, agonised boy and I wait, his dance of wracking pain goes on, minute after minute, maybe for five minutes. Then the door opens and we meet a wonderful man, he sees my boy, picks up the phone and relief is with us in a minute. He is kind and he is gentle and he understood in a micro second what my boy is going through. He hurries us through the admin procedures arranges more and stronger pain relievers, and he assures us that he can help us forward. He takes the boy away and he soon returns saying that we have to come back tomorrow when they will zap his cancer and that will ease the pain.

He takesk me aside and tells me that help is at hand and that he will arrange for us to see a palliative care consultant in a hospice near his home.

And so we drive home again, he had come through a trial, the like of which I had never witnessed, there was nothing I could imagine that could tear a human to shreds such as the pain of that day. But for now the race is over he is full of drugs and somehow awake, relieved, quiet; he has got through, but there remain the shadow that there will be more terrors ahead. We stopto eat some junk food, his appetite is immense, he gulps down his food like someone who is starved.

I deliver him to his mother, his sister is down after work. He is suddenly exhausted and we all help him into his downstairs bed. Things are rough; the reality of nursing at home hit us all, his mother is calm, his sister and daughter all very helpful, but the pain rages and he knows that he has to fight these demons alone. There are indignities, he can't piss into his bottle, he makes a mess, he is cross with himself. I watch hopelessly and try to ring the specialist sister from the hospital, I try a hundred times I never get through.

Another evening and another drive the fifty five miles home; I need to watch my tiredness, and more, the failing resilience of my spirit. For what I have witnessed this day had hurt me uncannily physically, I felt though I had been slammed in the guts with a baseball bat. I ache from head to foot. And then it hits me. What courage my boy had shown, when, after that dreadful interlude he sat quietly in the car; steeling himself toward the next, when the cancer will attack and devour him from within. He did not once query his fate, through those tranquil eyes he stared down the agonies of his future without one word of bitterness or complaint. So I had better pull myself together.

The next day I arrive for the journey back to the radiotherapy centre and learn that he has had a terrible night, but I also learn with great relief that other aid was at hand, the Macmillan nurse had come to supervise the ever changing medical supplies and prescriptions. The local pharmacy has laid on a daily delivery service, and the boy's doctor is keeping an eye. Suddenly we are not so alone and it makes a vast difference.

Today is much like yesterday though now we know our way and we arrive to more familiar surroundings..

Today he has more and better balanced drugs and he seems more resolved. Our discussion is about what we are doing today, why we are travelling these great distances back and forth – to make him more comfortable. Of all things in the world, he wants to be more comfortable, his focus is entirely on keeping these ferocious attacks at bay. It has become his purpose in life – not avoid dying but to be more comfortable.

I do not allow him to smoke in the car. He does not complain, but when we arrive at the hospital he darts off to have a fag while I park the car. I return to find him chatting to another ragged man. They seem at ease. He tells me the other bloke has a brain tumour and that he has only six weeks left. He is quietly composed and makes no comment about his comparative situation. He adds that the bloke who's got six weeks left said that the hospital had helped him, helped him a lot. "Good", is all I can think to say.

He goes for his radio zap, which doesn't take long- can't think why we didn't do it yesterday, another two hundred miles for a two minute treatment. There I go again , moaning about my lot. What a pig I can be.

We meet our hero, the Consultant and he chats and says he's fixed us up with a meeting with a palliative care consultant at a hospice near to my boy's home. He checks his patient's medicine requirements and arranges more drugs for us to take home. After such an efficient and expeditious treatment we wait an hour in the cheerless waiting room for news of the medicines. My boy goes out to smoke and meet some other patients most of whom are in a similar position to him. I ask about the medicine and we are directed to the hospital pharmacy that turns out to be a long way away. We trudge off and it is not long before my boy cannot walk. He rests and I scurry away and find a wheelchair. We make it to the pharmacy and collect the drugs. Our journey back to his home is quiet, we both anticipate tomorrow's meeting with the palliative care consultant with a mixture of hope and despair.

The meeting is set for tomorrow morning, "it's to make you more comfortable, to manage the pain." I insist. He nods, any help will do. He wants to get home and have some time with his pals. He wants to go out on his motorbike, he wants to feel the wind in his hair, he wants to laugh, share a joint and be free of pain.

We talk about his motorbike, how he did such wild things, how he and his pals sped down the autobahns of Germany at hair raising speeds. We laugh about the times he got in trouble because he looked like a what I call a beatnik – he laughs almost hysterically -shows how far I am from his culture. It dawns on me that he's not been just a useless miserable addict, an addict, true, but one with a life and his own joys and sorrows. He talks about his kids, they are still close to him, two daughters and a son who was sired by someone else. He has, despite all his trials, remained true to them, kept the faith with them. I feel uneasy and slightly ashamed.

I am beginning to recognise the pot holes in the road, I know the times when the rush hour will lengthen my journey, I tell myself I must use the journeys to think and hold the team together, I may have been a lousy father but now I know I must pay back for all those years of selfishness. I grieve for my son who is not yet dead. It hurts constantly as the miles roll on. When? How long? I know it's on everyone's mind but we dare not speak of it.

CHAPTER THREE

It's a bright sunny spring morning, my son and my daughter are together and off we go to the hospice to meet the palliative care consultant. The word hospice makes my son stiffen.

"I am not staying there," he says, before we've even left the end of the street. "Dad I am not staying there," he repeats firmly.

My mind is scrambled, he needs care, the sort we cannot give him at home. "Let's wait and see," I tell him, "let's wait and see."

"I'm not staying in there," he repeats. We drive on in silence.

The hospice is in a rural suburb of the city not far from the hospital where he'd suffered at the hands of the National Health Service. The shadow of the old experience falls upon us, and on him in particular. I drive quickly on and there it is, a lovely low rise building. It was built in light wood and soft silver metal frame. The lightness of it takes me by surprise, I don't know what to expect but whatever it is, this is not it. There is a beautiful sports car at the entrance which is a prize in a fundraising initiative for the hospice, my boy was momentarily diverted from his anxiety – it is an exotic speed machine and that is his thing.

Inside, the reception area is spacious and airy, there is literature everywhere, all of it about 'caring for life'. I check us in at the reception desk.

"What a lovely place," I venture.

"I am not staying here!" comes the adamant reply.

The light from a chapel shines onto where we sit, there is a lovely stained glass window. It is a place for peaceful contemplation, a place foreign to my boy who is not contemplative; I know he sees the place as a place where people die, where people prayed. He does not want to die, and despite his situation he doesn't want to pray either. His firm atheism surprises me, he makes no attempt to seek assurances for his afterlife. He is firmly without illusions of eternity, he is facing his end as a matter of fact.

My daughter and I exchange glances, and look away. Is there just the thought that we wanted to be rid of him? Pass our problem to someone else? I believe we both think the same thing and we both feel confused. Is it guilt or concern? We wait, and he becomes more anxious as the cancer started gnawing at him, I can see his eyes cloud and his face grimace and his body wrack. What can I do, what can his sister do? – just sit there and help him bear the pain. What's love all about?

Across the hall comes a tall young and pretty lady, I assume a volunteer. Her smile is radiant, she is slim tall and very attractive. She ignores me and goes straight to the patient and greets him warmly, "Sorry to keep you waiting, I'm the Palliative Care Consultant." She takes his hand calls him by his name and looks into his eyes. Then she turns and introduces herself to his sister and then to me. She beckons and we follow to an examination room where we sit, the three of us across a makeshift desk. Her eyes seldom leave my son, sometimes she asks his sister or me some questions, but her focus is on her patient. She takes him aside and examines him and slowly I see my boy give her his trust. Her voice, her expression, the extraordinary sensitivity is overwhelming. Together with our hero from radiology here is another saviour, someone who understands; who cares profoundly about my boy and about what he is going through. It is hard not to embrace her and break down. I can see my daughter feels the same.

It takes an hour of patient of careful analysis of his pain: Where? How often? On a scale of 1 to 10? Here? There? And so on. The patient, his sister and the Doctor work behind a screen, I can hear them clearly; the gentleness of the doctor's voice and the gathering confidence of my son's replies. I stand uselessly looking out the window. In addition I can hear the conversation about his drug habit, his needs and wants, it is now so matter of fact, there are no secrets any more.

At the end of the examination, we gather round the desk, and the doctor explains in great detail what she was all about. We all know the situation she says, and her job is to make my son as free from pain as possible. In this case she added there were special difficulties because my son has destroyed his venous system and she or anyone else would be unable to administer medicines intravenously, so there would have to be a period of observation and indeed experimentation with a cocktail of palliatives to see what would work best. The doctor felt that these exploratory efforts would be best done at the hospice.

"I am not coming in here to stay." The boy intervened. There was a short silence.

I put my hand gently on the back of his neck. "Let the doctor help you," I pleaded, he shrugged me off.

"I am not staying here," he repeated.

"This is not a long stay hospital, this is a place we get pain under control and then patients go home – patients here can go home whenever they like." The doctor's tone remains gentle and even. I feel desperation and confusion rise within me, my daughter sees my angst and beckons me to be still. I obey.

"Come," says the doctor, "Come and see some of the lovely rooms we have, one is reserved for you right now, come and see."

"I'm not staying in here."

"That's fine, no one will make you do anything, just come and see what lovely accommodation we have."

She leads the way through the sunny reception area, and down through broad light corridors on the other side of the building. The same light wood panels line the walls and the floor is beautifully carpeted, we pass children's play rooms, sitting rooms, coffee machines and little cafe rooms. We come to the centre of the complex; there was a light lounge area complete with piano opposite the working centre. It was quite busy, but everyone greets us and smile, and at the same time do not impose on my son's space. He is just another somebody to be welcomed and respected. It was uncanny how the warmth of welcome was balanced with respect, respect for my boy and respect for us all.

We look into a delightful room apparently reserved for my son if he so wishes. Again the walls were bright and what woodwork there was a was light oak, there was an entertainment centre that grabbed my boy's attention. There were patio doors that opened onto a private boardwalk terrace with table and chairs that overlooked a sweet duck pond and delightful garden.

"Well," said the doctor, "What do you think?"

"I'd rather be home," said my boy, with rather a softer tone.

"You sure?" I ventured, "it will only be for a while till they get you settled and then you can come home."

"Dad, I'd rather be home."

And so after a few formalities about arranging medicines through his local doctor, we make our way back to his home. There the house had already been transformed; the boy's bed had been rearranged and thoroughly cleaned, the little dining room been changed into a neat little bedroom.. His elder daughter was there to meet us and she and her father embrace, they clearly care for each other, and find comfort in each other's presence.

With typical lack of sensitivity I enquired whether the boy could climb the stairs and have a shower, and perhaps shave. The ladies of the house looked at me without comprehension. I shut up.

His daughter has arranged all the drug regime with time charts and measures so that the bewildering pile of medicines on the kitchen surface is put into some sort of system. Here is this young eighteen year old I hardly know imposing system where there could so easily be dangerous chaos.

The MacMillan nurse arrives and the army of women fuss and organise making me feel redundant. I am despatched to the local pharmacy to get more medicine, this turns out to be quite a chore and I have to hang around and go back and forth to the boy's doctor, prove my identity and all manner of other tasks because the medicine of such potency and quantities would be a God send to any illicit dealer. I do this with uncharacteristic patience, understanding perhaps for the first time how generous is the National Health Service in the UK. All this must have cost a fortune.

I do my duties and returned to the house where my boy seemed to have settled and is sleeping soundly. The ladies all agreed that tomorrow I am to have a day off, stay at home and keep in touch by phone. I kissed my sleeping son and drive away relieved; in the belief that the morning's session with the lovely lady doctor has somehow brought us some stable relief.

CHAPTER FOUR

It is hard to escape from someone else's precious last days. It is impossible to see the hours tick by and not be aware of time, now such a hard arbiter of life.

In my comfortable home, away from temporary bedrooms, piss bottles, and the shriek of someone else's pain, I am suspended in a miserable void that no end of kindness from my gentle wife can assuage. The Sunday newspaper holds no fascination, the ordinariness of the Sunday morning streets seem almost ghostlike. As I walk, I wonder how many other people are experiencing the horrors of losing their child. I wonder idly, as I walk each day, what's behind each door I pass on the neat estate on my way to pick up the paper. Behind each front door, is it a world of joy or pain? I see pensioners tend their gardens, relatives arrive for Sunday lunch. I see smiles, and hear children scream and laugh, and it all seems unreal. I have this great urge to stop and tell people about my boy. To tell them, - to tell them what? I don't know, but I am reminded that life goes on – here it is banal, ordinary and here am I; ordinary too.

I phone his home, he is settled he is sleeping, his daughter stayed with him all night, he's OK. Well not OK but he's fine don't worry – his pals are coming to see him – he wants to go out. I want to protest – go out? Are you crazy? If he wants to go out! – Why not? Yes – why not?

I put down the phone I am dumbfounded. My assumption has been and still is, that I must look after my boy, but that is clearly not his assumption. He wants to live his dream and that dream is not lying in his bed being cared for. I am not sure whether to be cross or to admit yet again that his mother knows him better, understands him better and loves him better than me. I cry quietly in my study I realise I do not want to share his last days with anyone and how selfish I am.

I speak to my daughter who visits him later in the day. She confirms he's been out with his pals but now has returned home exhausted. He is still eating like a horse and has lapsed back into sleep. "Dad, he's had a nice day." A nice day without me!

I sleep shallowly, my mind is numb, there is a part of me who wants to stay here, warm, with my lovely wife, and turn off the world. But I can't turn it off and the horrors of my boy's dilemma will not go away. It's early, the phone rings – I leap out of bed. It's his mother, the night has been hell. He's been in agony and the house is a shambles, his mother and his daughter have been up virtually all night. I ask a lot of stupid questions : Did you ring the doctor? Did anyone come? I don't hear any of her replies – she sounds tired and broken. I am on my way, unshaven and un-showered, I have no idea what I am supposed to do. I knife the car through the morning rush hour and arrive around eight. The neat little house is no more, it's stuffy, there are empty cups unwashed, my boy's bedroom is chaotic the floor is a mess. He is on the cross, he howls with pain. The whole house has been wrecked by the chaos of the suffering. It's as if a tornado of evil has swept through what was the neat little house.

His mother has aged, she is hurt, her back has been injured in the fray of the night. His young daughter looks exhausted and distressed. No child should witness this, or be asked to salve the impossible curse of this vicious evil disease.

The hospice is our only hope. I ring, there is some confusion, but soon a calm voice says, bring him to us, say ten o clock. Ten o'clock is still two dark hours away. I over rule his daughter and give him an extra large dose of his pain killer. Minutes pass, he is more tranquil, and says "sorry dad."

"Hang in, Boyo," I reply, "and don't be so bloody silly." He sleeps.

His mother's injury is real, she looks haggard and drawn, she cannot move. We make her comfortable, send for the doctor, and it is time to take my boy to the hospice. I wake him gently, we assemble his clothes and his medicines with all the notes and with some difficulty I put him in the car. He does not ask where we are going – so I tell him,

"We are going to where we can manage this pain." He says nothing.

It is a bright spring morning, we leave after rush hour and we arrive at our destination about ten minutes early. I stop at the entrance and drop him off, he can hardly stand, I think he will fall. I wave through the glass doors but no one sees. I leave the car there and rush in asking for a wheelchair. It materialises in seconds. There are few formalities, we have to sign in, now and on every visit, and sign out too. I wheel him down the corridors that seemed so welcoming last Saturday but now I am not sure of my way, I am not sure of myself, though my son is quiet and still in the chair.

We arrive at his room and we seem to have picked up a small crowd during our very short walk, the nurses (I presume they are nurses) gently and seamlessly take the chair from me, and welcome my boy to his new room. It's lovely and airy and the whole ambience is one of refreshing ease. They gently help him onto his bed, they call him by his name, they already seem to love him. I am stunned.

I sit, suddenly I remember the car is still outside the door, I explain and dart away to park. I am gone not five minutes. When I return there are two doctors at his bedside, I reverse out of his room, "No, no" they beckon, I sit listening as they gently explore the channels of his agony. It takes time, occasionally they ask me a question, I answer as best I can, becoming aware that I have not been with him through these most recent traumas.

The doctors finish, I follow them outside his room, I do not know what to say, I am tempted to ask, "how long?" – but I desist. The doctors walk away and then one turns and shakes my hand and tells me that my boy will be reviewed every day by a doctor, and his case will be discussed every day, and his medication will be reviewed every day until his pain is under control.

"You do understand," she adds, "that this is not long term care, as soon as your son is well enough he'll be able to go home."

"Well enough?" The astonishment in my voice is plain for all to hear.

"Yes," she repeats. "When his pain is controlled, he'll be able to go home."

I know, I am without medical knowledge, but what are we talking about? My boy well enough? They know and I know he's dying, so how can he be well enough to go home? Then it dawns on me what caring for life is about, it's about creating a quality of life no matter how short, so that life can be lived and enjoyed if even for only a minute, a day, or a year.

My boy is sleeping, a sweet young nurse tucks him in, she smiles at me, and says, "What do you think he'll like for lunch?" I choose lasagne followed by ice cream. She jots down my instructions and walks away with purpose. Five minutes later she's back, "let me show you around," she says.

My boy sleeps on, she touches my back, he'll be fine, we won't be long, and she ushers me on to my tour of this extraordinary place. I am introduced to people as we go, to cleaners, a man who describes himself as my son's batman, to nurses, to volunteers, I cannot tell who are staff and who are volunteers. They all wear tags but they all seem entirely engrossed in doing what they are doing. I see a lot but take very little in.

After my tour that included guest bedrooms, coffee lounges, and family rooms I am taken back to him, he is still sleeping. I sit and watch him sleep, his breath is regular but he sometime winces in his sleep. I wander out on to his screened patio/boardwalk, it has a table and chairs and overlooks the delightful duck pond and garden. There are other visitors and patients, sitting out in the sun, it could be a Centre Park, it is serene and beautiful and it is populated by people who are at ease, and if I look closely, many are in easy animated conversation, many smile and laugh. I sit near the door where I can see my boy, I feel the sun on my face and for the first time in weeks I feel a small sense of respite. I phone his Mum and his sister and I tell them that he is in the most wonderful care.

He wakes and has a drink; a nurse comes and checks him over. He declares he's already feeling better. The bed is comfortable, he feels rested. He gets up and we walk out onto his patio and we sit watching the ducks. He smiles and says what a lovely place this is. He lights a cigarette, I huff, he smiles even chuckles. "What's the point, Dad." Indeed what's the point?

I find it hard not to hate the idea of tobacco and cigarettes. The sight and smell of them raise in me a reflex of disgust and loathing. I don't know what the drugs did to him but I know that tobacco is killing him, but deep down I know that I smoked from an impossibly young age and only gave them up when I had a stroke more than twenty years ago. But tobacco makes me angry.

Lunchtime comes and he piles into his lunch, served on the patio with a huge smile by one of the nurses, who on departure sweeps away the ashtray. I can't resist a nasty comment about cigarettes, she gently berates me.

"Never mind your dad," she says to him. "How are you feeling."

He barely hears her, he is devouring his lunch; I am astonished at the speed he eats. I am slightly alarmed that his appetite is so voracious. His table manners, where are they? I remain rooted in my own world when it is plain he is no longer there, whatever drives him whether spiritual or physical, he is playing to different rules. These rules are hard to divine, and even harder to understand, but I begin to understand for the first time that I cannot assume anything, what he's thinking or feeling, I can only do my best to care for what life he has left.

We've only been in this place half a day, and I've learned so much. It's as if that in his suffering and his situation, there is another dimension, I can sense it but not experience it; but at least I am aware of it. I know that for some time I have studiously avoided discussing the future, but the dilemma is greater than simply that. It is a question of living in the moment and cherishing each one as eternal. This sounds pretentious, but it makes sense to me, and the thought defines what it is I can do for my boy. These people in this wonderful hospice understand this, and their 'strap line'; "Caring for life" is what they are all about. To do this is beyond most of us. Yet here is a team of diverse but devoted people, who care for the fragments of terminally ill people's lives, and together generate such a generosity of spirit that is truly in another dimension from everyday life.

He has another cigarette, I contain my bile, and we talk about motorbikes. He tells me things I never knew, about bikes and speeds, and adventures. He tells me about his friends who are materially successful, and those he loves. He talks of those who've been good to him and those who've been even wilder than him. He paints a picture, there are few dark corners as he sees it, and I do not pry.

He is tired and retires to his bed, he is suffering again. I call the nurse who comes in a trice. She asks about the pain, its location, its strength and its character. A minute passes and soon palliative drink is administered and he sleeps once more. I walk into the sun and talk to the ducks.

The afternoon ticks by, I read my paper, walk in the garden and keep returning to his room, but he sleeps peacefully. The afternoon ebbs away and my daughter and his daughter arrive.

I do not know my granddaughter who calls me Grandpa. I find it strange and a bit uncomfortable. When the boy wakes he embraces his daughter, there is deep affection, unfettered and honest. I feel a bit ashamed. It is plain that they have enjoyed a long, continuous and close relationship. They have done this out of my sight and beyond my caring, no wonder I feel sad and confused.

They, father and daughter, go out onto the patio and roll cigarettes and light up. I can't stop myself from incandescing: How can she smoke when she's sharing this experience? How can he let her smoke when he's dying in this ghastly way?

I involuntarily go into a rant about tobacco and its dangers. I am haranguing them.

"Dad, it doesn't matter, I can't tell her to stop when I enjoy my fags."

Should I challenge him? Shall I tell him, 'grow up son and do something responsible for once in your life!' I keep quiet.

"I'll give up, Grandpa I promise, but not now."

"Don't give up smoking, give up your next cigarette, that's all you have to do," I plead.

I back off, who wants conflict here? But I still seethe with anger. Can't they see?. I know he's dying, I know he likes cigarettes, but can't he try and help his daughter break the habit we know to be so lethal? I think of an ancient James Cagney picture where the brutal villain goes to the electric chair, feigning cowardice so that he will discourage his followers from evil.

I am disconsolate because to fight will be wrong, and to acquiesce is also wrong. There is nothing here that is right, his situation, our history, my relationship with my granddaughter – it's all wrong, except that I know I love my son, and I know he trusts me, I think and I hope that he loves me.

He also embraces his sister. My lovely daughter, again there is a familiarity that I can only hope to acquire.

I escape to the refreshment room to make tea. It has been a long day, I am exhausted. I know the girls have been to work and college; they too must feel the strain. I must go, I have sixty long miles home, and I must be alone to purge the discord that grinds uncomfortably between my love, grief and confusion.

CHAPTER FIVE

At something past ten o'clock in the morning, I arrive at the hospice, the car park is almost full. I wonder how many people are involved here. Patients and their families, employees, volunteers, there seem to be a lot. I buzz the intercom and I sign in. The lady at reception is not someone I've seen before and I am disappointed, despite her charm. I want to see people I recognise; I want to be familiar with everyone and everything.

I go urgently to my son's room, and again there is someone I do not recognise at his bedside. He is a doctor, he wields a stethoscope writes into a patient's note file. He is talking to my boy quietly. He barely acknowledges my arrival, he beckons me to sit. He is a big man, about fifty five. He has a very large balding head, wears lightly framed glasses and radiates concentration and concern. His face is solid and open, he looks the picture of health. He has not spoken to me yet, but already I am impressed. I instantly trust him. He continues his examination of my son, in the midst of the questions about pain, he asks within my earshot, "Is this your Dad?" He acknowledges me with a tiny wave of his hand. He continues his careful work, I sit watching, listening in silence. Eventually he is finished.

He introduces himself, shakes my hand solidly, he is the Medical Director. He explains he wasn't in yesterday when my boy arrived, he is 'matter of fact', yet concerned; steering a wise and sure course over the bumpy road of the dying and the incurable. He tells me my boy is in a very difficult condition because he cannot accept intravenous infusions. He explains, something I can barely understand, that as the cancer tightens its grip, his brain will be flooded with calcium, and the only way to effectively inhibit this is by intravenous infusion. They will work on alternatives but it will not be easy. He pats me on the shoulder.

I am bursting with questions, what does all this mean? Calcium, what will be the consequences? Can he help the pain? Is he my son's messiah? How Long? How Long, is always the guilty question. He explains at length the calcium issue, in short it will make what future my son has harder, it will make his last days less lucid, and he will become more disoriented as things break down as they must. I beg within, that this must not come to pass, but I know it must, and I trust this doctor absolutely. He is preparing me for more agonies ahead. He assures me that he and his team will do all in their powers to make my boy's journey as easy as they can. Despite the fear, I am comforted, for the medical director talks to me so directly and at the same time so sympathetically that he makes me feel he shares my burden.

He tells me that he recognises the suffering of relatives as well as his patients, and emphasises that his team is here for us all. I am moved to weep again, I thank him; mumbling I go back to my son's room. I did not ask the question 'When?'

My son is sitting up, he is chipper, "Hello, Dad." He greets me with a smile. "I'm feeling a lot better, I'll be home again before you can say knife!"

"Good boy, that's the spirit," I'm still choking back the tears, "but patients must be patient. Give these guys time to settle down the pain and we'll have you home in no time."

We walk to his terrace and he rolls a fag, lights up and begins a discourse on the sexual habits of the wild ducks that populate the duck pond. We laugh and walk gently around the pond and into the garden. It is a lovely April morning, we talk easily about all sorts of things, I find myself hanging on his every word. Our idyll is broken when suddenly I see he can go no further; we've walked about a hundred yards. He sits to rest on a bench and we talk some more, we are both aware of his infirmity, and how fragile the moment is. There are to be many more moments such as this one, all beautiful and precious minutes where father and son are at ease with one another. In those eternal loving moments, each caring unconditionally for one another, these are perhaps amongst the sweetest moments of my life.

After a considerable rest we stroll back the hundred yards through the flowers stopping every ten yards or so pretending to admire them. We make it back to his terrace, he is exhausted. I help him back into bed and he immediately falls asleep. I am so pleased to see him with less pain, I am elated, I phone everyone to tell them how much better he is.

I watch him sleep; he is more serene than I have seen him for weeks. This is a good day; I stand at his bed, and stroke his brow. It is damp, with sweat, and I see my forty one year old boy, gaunt and grey, looking nearer seventy. This emaciated wreck is my boy – oh! I should have loved him more.

Eventually he wakes and he expresses his hunger, "He's starving." Once more he wolfs down his lunch with alarming speed. He tells me he'd like some ginger beer, so off I go and search the locality for a convenience store. I get lost and can't find my way back to the hospice. I feel disoriented and cross, I drive very quickly, I am talking to myself, I am behaving irrationally. I stop and ask a pretty young mum wheeling a pram, the way back. She is sweetly precise and in minutes I know where I am and cool down.

When I get back to his room my daughter and his two daughters are sitting round his bed. They are chatting twenty to the dozen. I unload my purchases that include not only ginger beer but a large miscellany of confectionery. He immediately shares the new found bounty with his daughters.

They are nice girls, at least they present themselves as nice girls, they are eighteen and sixteen. The elder is tall and rangy with a pretty freckled face and short tomboyish hair. Her younger sister is blonde with bright cheeks. I note the younger one bites her nails. After doing serious damage to the confectionery supply my son and his brood wander onto the patio and they all light up their rolled cigarettes. I half heartedly launch my anti-smoking tirade but my daughter intervenes, "Give it a rest Dad." I puff my disapproval.

My daughter and I leave him and his brood wittering away. We walk in the garden and talk about his future. We talk about his daughters, I am lost as to know what to do, or say to them. Do they appreciate the situation? The elder child has been very brave and adult and the younger seems detached even aloof; as if all this is nothing to do with her.

I am afraid that my boy will ask me to look after his girls. I don't know if I've got enough love in me. Besides I hardly know them, when my boy announced the pregnancy of his then girlfriend so long ago, I was shocked, I had never met the lady, and when I did I have to say I was less than impressed. However I played the honourable father of the father of the child to be. I gave my advice, which everyone ignored, and the baby was duly born. That birth was followed by another, some two years later. My boy got a house on the local authority that seemed very pleasant and there his family lived as far as I knew happily, but not for ever after. After ten years of their partnership the mother and children disappeared back to the maternal grandma's home, and I seldom saw them again, though my boy kept in constant touch. The girls had grown up without a grandfather, and the grandfather didn't much care. We shared very little, the girls never came to my home. I sent checks on birthdays and Christmas at the behest of my wife of the time.

Now here we all are; thrown together in the tragedy that is my boy. Knowing what I know now, about his addiction and drug taking I am more confused than ever about how these girls must have been brought up. It occurs to me that my boy and his mate must have been complicit in drug abuse. What must these two children have been through? Yet there is this unmistakable affection and filial love, so whatever the horrors of drug abuse their relationship has survived and even flourished. I catch a glimpse of my own revealed experience, that despite everything I love my boy; come what may!

That afternoon I agree to drop the two girls off at their home some twenty miles or so on my way home. It is not long before the elder asks me directly, "What do the doctors say Grandpa, is Dad going to be alright? Please please tell us," she complains. "Nobody will tell us anything."

Is this my responsibility? I drive on for a moment or two, and then I do my best. "Your Dad is very sick, he has cancer, he is not going to get better." I swiftly add, "We must all try and make him comfortable..." I was going to say, "While he's still with us." But I don't.

There is silence in the back of the car, and then the tremulous voice of the younger girl; "Grandpa, is Daddy going to die?"

"We're all going to die sweetheart, but yes your Dad is going to die."

I hear them sniffle as they try to contain their tears. "When, Grandpa, when will Dad die?"

"My dears, it's impossible to say, perhaps a year perhaps sooner but really no one really knows." I want to stop the car and give them a hug, but motorways are not places for sentiment "We must all be brave and love your dad. If you need anything, please get hold of me ..." What humbug!

CHAPTER SIX

Another day, another journey over the familiar pot holes at break-neck speed. My wife has not once queried my reckless schedule, she has gently suggested I go a little later, perhaps take a day off. I hear her, but only just. She travels with me once or twice, but it's hard for her and I know that my boy and me, we're getting to be an exclusive couple, so she sits patiently but outside.

I am afraid, that if I miss a moment, I will forever regret it. I had planned to spend the weekend away in York on some writer's junket, should I go? I spent a lot of money on it – I don't know what I will do. If I knew when? If I knew when, I could be sure to be with him, I could prepare everyone. I determine that I must ask, - I must ask.

My son has had a bad night, compared with yesterday, he looks appalling. Just like the day when we went to the hospital for his radiotherapy. His nurse is with him, she smiles, she is holding his hand. The doctor has been, she tells me and they've just administered another palliative, hopefully he'll be more comfortable soon. My guts wrench, I hold his spare hand, he barely notices me, I resist my urge to scream, to try to exorcise this beast. I shut my eyes tightly; I want to resist the tears but they roll, hot, down my face.

It is hard not to shout obscenities, it's really what I want to do, my anger and frustration is overwhelming me. I hear myself sobbing and have to leave the room. I sit in the coffee room and wipe my tears, and for want of anything else make a coffee. I am intent on doing that simple thing, I do not notice the young lady nurse, someone I have never seen before, coming in. She strokes my back, I turn and she holds me, just for a second. I straighten up and apologise.

"What for?" she says.

"For assaulting a beautiful young lady I've never met before." I try to smile. She's already on her way out the door. She tells me her name and she disappears down the corridor. I talk to myself, I must get a grip, a deep breath and I go back to his room. He is asleep.

I am preoccupied about going to York, despite all that's happening I feel a nagging desire to get on with my life. I argue that I am selfish and lacking the guts to give everything to my boy. Perhaps there lurks a sign of hopelessness, of giving up. Everyone advises me to go to York, what difference, they ask, can I make? This hurts; I thought I was making a difference. Today hope has been dashed in that I expected the hospice to deliver an improvement; it has been only three days since he was admitted. The promise of the first two days has been ruined by this morning's set back. It's like a brutal boxing match, you win some rounds and you lose some, the difference is you know it's going to end in a knock out; we are going to lose, whatever.

I watch him sleep, he seems less restless, perhaps this mornings review has got him back on track to a few days of reasonable comfort. I anticipate his waking and wonder what it will be like. Will he be more comfortable? Will he still be in agony? I am anxious and afraid. My watch tells me it's still early, I fidget, try to read my newspaper but cannot concentrate. I want to leave the room but I do not want my boy to wake up alone, so I stay. I doze and dream about all the wonderful things, not least my daughter, his sister. How sweet and kind she is. How patient and kind, how calm and reliable. Of all this woe, there is at least this great gift, a daughter who is everything I could ask for, and more. And then there are my granddaughters, I have this chance to get to know them. I am happy to see that their relationship with their father is so affectionate. The older girl is impressive; she's shown strength of character and courage beyond her years. What next for them? What next for us?

I am woken from my reverie as I catch sight of the Medical Director passing the open door. I race after him, slow to a walk and ask timorously if I may have a word.

We sit in the comfortable lounge area, he waits for me to start. I don't know what to say, well I do, but I am afraid to ask the question; "How Long?"

The Medical Director asks me about my boys' hands and fingers. I have long noticed that his fingers are misshapen and that the ends of his fingers are spoon like enlarged at the finger tips, His fingernails are huge almost claw like, but this I recall is not new, it may be to do with his occupation, dealing with cements and plasters, or indeed it may have been a result of drug abuse, all I know is he's been like this for a very long time. The Medical Director I think is interested purely out of professional curiosity. Then there is an awkward silence, so I blunder in;

"He obviously had a lousy night," I say, "Will he settle down?"

"Your son is very ill, and we are doing all we can to make him comfortable, but you need to understand this is not a simple thing." I nod. "We are trying to develop a cocktail of palliative medicines that will make him more comfortable, but in this particular case and because of his history it is both difficult and complex. We know how you feel," he smiled, "Watching your loved one suffer is horrendous and we are conscious of your suffering too, but you have to believe that we are doing all we can."

He went on, and I felt so grateful for his time and his kindness it didn't matter that I did not follow all the detail. He gave me hope that my boy could still be stabilised to enjoy perhaps a short period at home.

Then I said it, I asked the unaskable, "How long do you think he has left?"

He held me in his gaze. "I understand why you want to know," he smiled a winsome smile. "It is very hard to tell, but I should have thought that if we measure time by days, weeks, months and years, I think we'd be talking weeks."

"He does not want to know," I blurted, "My boy definitely does not want to know!".

"Have no fear he will not learn from us."

"Thank you, you are very kind." I began to weep uncontrollably.

He patted my shoulder, "You must rest and keep yourself strong, there is time yet, so take some time for yourself to rest, have some time off. We will keep in touch day and night, never fear my friend, look after yourself you will need all the strength you can muster, but when I said weeks, it could be many weeks, but weeks not a week so look after yourself." He got up to go. "Anything else you want to know?"

"No thank you," I replied, blowing my nose and mopping my tears.

I go back to my son's room. He is awake. "Hi Dad," he says. "Could you get me a cuppa tea?"

"Sure thing. How are you feeling?"

"Better thanks, had a shitty night, but I feel much better now."

"Good Boy, just a jiffy and I'll get the tea." My spirit soars, it is astonishing how I swing so quickly from despair to euphoria. If he's this good tomorrow I shall go to York.

I get back to his room, he is outside he is having a cigarette. It is a lovely day, he tells me he is hungry and looking forward to lunch. We have a fifty yard walk, it is wonderful. He again regales me with tales of the sexual habits of the wild ducks. We laugh together, yes, it is wonderful.

During the annihilation of a very substantial lunch he tells me that if he feels this well he'll want to go home soon. I do not disagree. I talk to the nurse, the lovely jolly plump one, and she says he has to be stable in terms of serious pain for forty eight hours and then they will be happy to see him go home. Spirits are high.

I am conscious of the knowledge that has been shared with me – Weeks! What do I do with it? With whom do I share it? Weeks – how many weeks? This awful knowledge claws at the joy of seeing him with less pain, despite the knowledge, I am at a loss. My mind is numbed that he will so soon be gone, I hold his hand and we enjoy an hour before I have to go, it is hard to hide my grief.

I try to think what 'weeks' means. It's not months, but it might be more than one month. It's an analysis that my training will not let me escape. I know I need more information, more certainty, but I know there is no such thing. I question my own reason for wanting to know, there seems nothing but confusion. If the hospice is thinking of letting my boy go home and I am fairly certain they are, then I surmise that he has between three and eight weeks left. I can barely breathe as I take in my own reasoning, I feel physically sick. I excuse myself from my boy's room and sit alone in the lounge resplendent with its baby grand piano. A volunteer is playing, songs from the shows, he plays very well, I envy him his talent and his evident cheerfulness. I feel very lonely for the first time since this ordeal began. I am desolate now that the ultimate goodbye is so close. How will he be; my boy? He's been so brave till now, and he's getting all the help that's possible; but soon, so soon, he will die.

I approach a nurse who we have come to know so well. I tell her what I know. She nods in consent to the prognosis. I ask what will happen. She tells me that they will try to stabilize his suffering and they still aspire to send him home, but that was still some time away, but the last twenty four hours had shown promise, but forty eight hours pain free was the bottom line, and then he can go home. I remark on his eating so heartily. Yes she concurs, when he loses his appetite she says, then that will signal a new phase. I do not ask what that phase will be, I know, and I call it the 'last lap', and it will come, I know, soon enough.

I wait for my daughter to arrive after her work. She looks tired, but she smiles and kisses her sleeping brother. I take her outside and share my awful knowledge, she is remarkably calm, I feel she is holding back to support me . We embrace and we cry in unison, her succour is beyond anything I have ever valued, she holds me up as the song goes, she really does, and I feel better, stronger and more balanced. We compose ourselves and discuss what to say to his mother, what not to say to his children. She tells me how dreadful I look and that I must rest – Go to York! Get away, take a break! She commands. On the weekend there will be no shortage of visitors, the children, his mum, my daughter and doubtless some of his friends. I am still in two minds, I put off a decision till tomorrow.

On my way home I visit his mother, the cavalry has arrived in the shape of her sister, a sensible, intelligent and capable woman for whom I have much respect and affection. I have not seen her for many years. My former wife is still unwell but the house has been restored to its usual tidiness. After a brief greeting I tell my boy's mother what I know. She wails a sad and heart rending cry and then weeps. I hold her gently, I say nothing, there is nothing more to be said.

She asks, "When can I have him home?" Despite the chaos of last week she has no hesitation, she wants him home. I am moved by the generosity of her spirit, she has been through untold tortures so recently, and yet there is no hesitation, she wants him home.

CHAPTER SEVEN

It's my last visit of the week I have been persuaded that I should go to York.

My boy is so-so, not without pain but certainly more settled than he has been. The Medical Director is optimistic that he can go home next week. He adds a cautionary note that he can't promise anything but he felt they were making progress.

I am cheerful, and so is the patient, the lovely spring weather is sustaining its own glory, the garden is blooming and the ducks having a wonderfully promiscuous time. My son wants to get out of here, I can see the light is back in his eyes, our conversation is light and positive. We talk about the weather prospects for his homecoming, as if we are planning a vacation. I suppose we are, his last few days or weeks of enjoying his friends and family. Yet again the joy of his relief from pain is tempered by the inevitable march of time. He is noticeably stronger and our walk round the pond goes well, I measure and compare how many yards he can cover without a rest. I measure in steps, I remember what flower was near where we stopped yesterday, a yard more is a small triumph, this small step is a measure of how we care for him and how much he can enjoy what's left.

Once more I am so grateful for the fantastic care that he is receiving; these lovely people are making his remaining life bearable. They all, every one of them, knows why they do what they do. Each and everyone is devoted to my son and all the other patients. These are not the guardians of the hopeless they are the custodians of the spark of life; I am in awe of them.

As is usual, my boy is tired after his walk so he lays

down on his bed, but on this occasion he does not drop off to sleep. He asks for a cup of tea, so I dutifully toddle off to make us both a cuppa. As I return I meet the chaplain at his door. He is a jolly fellow, bearded and rotund. "I've come to see your son" he says, "may I come in?" I lead the way. The chaplain carries a Bible under his arm.

My son becomes agitated. He summons me to his bedside. He whispers in a rather loud stage whisper, "Tell him to go away, I don't want to talk to him."

I am surprised and embarrassed. I turn to the chaplain, and relay my son's missive, "I'm sorry," I say, "He doesn't want to talk to you."

The chaplain, says he understands and that he will be available for anything at any time, for patient or relative. I apologise once more and suggest that perhaps he try another time. My boy reiterates quite loudly this time that he does not want to see the chaplain at all. I shrug my shoulders, what else can I do. The chaplain apologises for intruding and for carrying his Bible, the Bible he says sometimes puts people off. He assures me and the boy that the Bible is not a necessary accoutrement and that he is always available for a chat. Loudly from the bed come the unmistakable words of dismissal to the chaplain. I am shocked but the chaplain takes the hint and exits without further ado. I feel sorry for the chaplain, and feel inclined to admonish my boy, I sigh and sit- there are so many things I don't know, or understand.

I am about to start a conversation, but when I look at him, he is asleep.

I am troubled by his rejection of the chaplain on two grounds, firstly I thought he was rude, and secondly and much more importantly he seems to remain adamant about his death being –The End. I can understand agnosticism, I can understand cynicism, but I find it hard to accept the desolation of absolute atheism. He appears to want to go to his end without hope. I am much saddened by this, and in the silence of my quiet reverie, I am glad I did not challenge him. I am very weary of discussing the matter at all. The last thing I want to do is upset what equilibrium remains, if he has certain mindsets then so be it, but in the context of our family, as much as that exists, it has been firmly based on the christian perspective.

In earlier bleak days of loss I had found the christian community a great help to me, and although my boy has obviously been estranged from any sort of church for many years I somehow expected him to welcome some spiritual nurturing at this time when he knows beyond all doubt that his end is nigh.

I have certainly prayed for him, for his deliverance, for this cup to pass, for help. And I suppose the only prayer that was answered was this place and its people. My own faith in retrospect seems flaky, driven in times of need and forgotten in times of plenty. The God and redeemer I believed in, I treated like a servant or a genie in a bottle; to be summoned when times were difficult. Perhaps my boy is right after all, my God of mercy hasn't been particularly lenient of his treatment of my boy. All nonsense I know, but still, my son's legacy to me, might be a need to reflect on many things, not least my faith or lack of it.

As if there is an alarm in his being my boy wakes promptly at lunch time, he is famished, raises himself from his bed, shoos away my attempts to help him, puts on his dressing gown and walks steadily onto the patio where he settles and rolls another cigarette. I cannot help but smile, he's so much better today, he radiates happiness, yes – happiness, bizarre as that may sound. A nurse appears to see if he is ready for lunch, I have not seen her before but my son recognises her from his childhood. They chat happily about times gone by and their common acquaintances from yore. The conversation is not marred by pain nor pity or self-consciousness. It is extraordinary in its ordinariness, two old friends chatting after a chance meeting. "It's great to see you," remarks my son. "Lovely to see you too," the nurse replies, "we can have a chat later I must get your dinner."

As usual the substantial meal is wolfed down in quick time, and we enjoy a cup of tea in the sunshine. I am struck by the miraculous gift of such a lively day, if only it can be sustained – if only? He has another cigarette; we talk idly about his children and his aspiration for them. I remain unsure, I have no idea what to say, though I feel the pressure to promise I will oversee their future, but deep down I have serious doubts. Soon he is weary and it is time for his afternoon nap.

I meander into the centre of the complex, and I see his school time friend, she comes over to me, "I'm so sorry to see him here," she says. "He was such a lovely boy- everybody liked him, he was just a great kid."

I thank her. "I know," I say, but do I, and did I really? She chats a little more and for the first time I see the professional poise slip. I see a tear in her eye, "I must go I have things to do." She turns and marches smartly away.

My daughter, his daughter, his mother and her sister all arrive almost at once. I am glad to see them and tell them about what a good day it's been. The patient still sleeps, so they all assemble on the patio all whispering and waiting for him to wake. When he does, I feel the space is very crowded, I mutter my excuses, say farewell to my boy, I will not see him for three days. I leave, feeling afraid, and sad and elated.

CHAPTER EIGHT

The following morning I set out for York having made several telephone calls; most of them unnecessary, I am unable to relax – after several weeks of daily visits I have become obsessed with the fear that I will miss a moment and live to regret it. Yet there have been so many days when I've just sat by his bedside while he sleeps. When he sleeps I watch for restlessness, the signs of a troubled mind, of nightmares and of panic. For the most part since he's been in the hospice his sleep has looked to me, deep and peaceful. Even these quiet times are precious, when he appears to be without pain and soundly asleep and at peace.

My wife who has patiently allowed me to have my own space over these last weeks bids me farewell, "Don't worry," she says, "everything will be fine. Relax! The conference will take your mind off things – enjoy yourself."

Now as the miles whip by, I am driving ever further away from him, I try to stay calm but there's a nagging angst that I am doing the wrong thing. I am hungry and I stop at a service station outside York, it is bedlam, all families on their way to spring holidays. I am conspicuous as a single male. After a tentative look into the eateries, I retreat, I don't have the confidence to wade into the fray of all these holiday makers. My reticence conquers my hunger, so I continue my journey – I am very hungry.

I find my way to the university campus which is very handsome, there are hordes of aspiring authors registering, the queues are long and the organisers not very organised. When I get to the front I find I have no badge, so I am directed to a side office where a young man fusses and eventually prints me off my badge and pass. I find I am billeted on the other side of the campus and I manoeuvre my car around the site avoiding no parking zones that appear to be everywhere. I am misdirected at least twice and I feel mightily depressed, the map I have been given makes little sense, I eventually park where I think is near my room, only to find it's a half mile walk to the allotted student residence. I unpack, gather my papers and set off across the site to join the first conference session. I phone the hospice as I walk; all is well, my boy has a room full of visitors.

The campus is situated around a hexagonal lake, the lake is full of wildlife, there are a number of willow trees that soften the hard lines of the modern functional architecture. It works aesthetically in this spring weather the scene is pleasant on the eye, it must be a great place to be at university.

The ducks seem as promiscuous here as at the hospice, I smile ruefully I hope that the sunny day there is not scarred with pain. The university buildings are baffling as I am now quite ancient and my ability to assimilate new places and faces is noticeably diminished. I have to admit that I've lost confidence. I approach the melee with trepidation, and note with some dismay that I am not only older than the majority but possibly the oldest man in the huge room.

Suddenly there is a spontaneous movement and the crowd disperses like ants each delegate rushing purposefully to his or her allotted session. The majority are female and in their early middle age. They are all earnest and enthusiastic, they move with an air of confidence. It strikes me that the Seminar entitled – "How to get published" ought to be sparsely populated since the degree of plain self confidence and assurance is overwhelming. I creep into the lecture theatre that has taken me ten minutes to find, hence my late self conscious and noisy entry. I should be wearing sneakers or trainers not my heavy brogues, but then perhaps I ought not to be here at all.

I listen to a charming young lady apparently a hugely (at least published author) successful writer, who writes I gather about love affairs between women or at least that's her subject when at last I net into the session. The presenter who talks well, comes to an end of her presentation in minutes, the rest of the session is devoted to questions and hopefully useful answers. I muse that it is a good wheeze to get paid, say very little and then take questions. When my paying guests used to come to listen to me, I laboured under the illusion that I had to bone up meticulously on my subject and give a word perfect presentation, and then expect questions – this lady was obviously smarter than me.

Nor was I used to the informality hence the brogues versus the trainers. Still my five hundred quid had been invested and I should try to get something in return. So I spent the day desperately trying to get to impossibly coded conference locations. It occurred to me that they gave degrees here in all likelihood for those who found their way to the appropriate lectures. At first if you are never late, and honours if you sat in English language lectures when you'd set out to do Chemistry. All the billowing skirts and flying scarves gave the place an air of Marks and Spencer's. The women chatted to everyone and the male delegates were noticeably more reticent, so there is a constant high pitch rather like being a delegate to a WI meeting. Many of the delegates were arty crafty and dressed in what I consider bizarre fashion; huge necklaces, massive collections of rings on their fingers, and giant pieces of metal round their wrists, somewhat reminiscent of Star wars; I imagined them clanking away at their computers.

At meal times I tried to sidle up to fellow delegates, begin a conversation and hopefully follow the unfortunate to a table and thus have an avenue of security, it is so much worse when I staggered from table to table, holding my lunch tray aloft and seeking a spare seat, and being told as often as not, that the seat was taken already. I have managed to find a few kind souls, both male and female and I have studiously avoided discussing the Elephant in my room, I don't know how long I can do this. At each break I rush out and telephone for updates on my boy's current state of wellbeing.

There are highlights, there are celebrities – though none that I recognise nor in most cases have heard of. The lectures are all about slush piles, agents' whims, How to get an agent, do you need an agent? What makes a good agent, electronic publishing, writing courses, successes and failures too. There are sessions where brave authors read their work, there is a jolly dinner and plenty to drink – this is my forte, here I am comfortable. The highlight is an interview with an agent or reader who has read my stuff. I am told gently but firmly that my writing is OK but the book is hopeless. I am disappointed but not surprised, I had great reservations about it anyway, it was my attempt to write a popular novel, and if I learn anything here it's that I'm as far adrift of popular culture as it is possible to be.

CHAPTER NINE

The break was over, I return from York with little enthusiasm for my writing career. My score of four books and collected poetry is of no importance; now, even less so. My boy is what is important now, I must lay aside all other things, the clock ticks on, his time is slipping through the fingers of life and soon he will be gone. I am impatient to see him. I am informed that things have gone well and that it is likely – barring disaster- that he will be allowed home - soon – very soon. Even tomorrow.

I am at the hospice, I am comfortable, I am glad to be here, I know this place; it is a place, an institution and the home of hope that cares for life. My son is sitting up, the Medical Director and a colleague are with him. I have not seen him for days, I am rudely reminded how sick he is. His cheeks are sunken, his arms like bleached twigs, but his eyes are still alight. He sees me and smiles, there is in his smile a small flame of warmth, he is glad to see me. I resist the urge to hug him, instead I gently take his skeletal head and kiss his damp brow, it is so good to be with him.

It is planned that he will come home tomorrow, but first he must go to the hospital for x-rays on his leg, the one ulcerated and weeping. Yes of course I will take him after lunch.

The doctors leave us alone, my boy talks about his children. I mutter in response because I don't know them nor do I want to make any promises I may not keep. His love for them is palpable; I am unable to share his aspirations and his recollections. He wants to leave what meagre estate he has to them. What estate? I hear you ask. Well since his illness we have, collectively, his mother and I, applied for social support, which my son never had. In truth he owes his mother a great deal more than the State paid out. However we feel he should keep what money there is , so that he has some small amount to leave to whom he chooses. I am a little sad that he does not think of all the support he has had from his mother for years. She has fed him and sheltered him for a long time, many years, and he in his addiction paid her not a penny. Still this is not the time for recrimination. He asks that I will help. I say of course I will do what I can. I think he knows my uncertainty; he lets me off the hook.

The day follows its usual ritual, a walk, a sleep an attack on lunch then more sleep. But today we have the journey to the hospital for x-rays on his leg. There is part of me that wonders – why bother? However the prospect of hope, however small, is a great driver.

The journey to the hospital is short, and it holds uncomfortable memories for us both. The place is modern and I assume built to accommodate the traffic of the buses and hundreds of cars and ambulances that traversed the site. It is in a permanent state of chaos, fortunately I know my way around, but despite this I struggle with the conflicts of parking, getting a wheelchair and not leaving my boy unattended, though he is quite content to join the hapless bunch of smokers at the hospital entrance. So the situation dictates what I do;drop him off with the hapless hopeless smokers and go away to find a parking space that can take anything up to twenty minutes which in this case it does.

I return; hunt for a wheelchair and start my search for the X-ray department through the maze of anonymous corridors and along many yards of polished floors, following signs that are multicoloured and confusing. We find the X-ray department and to our dismay discover that the waiting room is packed, not only is it packed it is very cramped with little room for manipulating a wheel chair and less still a wheelchair with my son's sorely damaged leg protruding. I park him in the corridor and lodge his papers with the department reception. We settle down to wait. We are both content to let the tide of progress take its time. I am weary after all the pushing and shoving, but have nowhere to sit. My son sees my discomfort and tells me to go inside and find a seat in the waiting room, eventually I do, right by the door so I can keep an eye on my boy. Eventually his name is called and I steer him into the X-ray studio. They are mercifully quick and we are out in minutes. The results of the X-ray will take a day or two to get back to the hospice. I wonder once more – what's the point?

On the way back my son's spirits are high, he is excited about going home, he tells me all the things he's going to do. His expectations seem to be fantasy but I encourage him, simultaneously advising patience and some care. He says; "Dad, let me be... right?" I nod, I have no idea what I've agreed to.

I visit his mother, all is prepared for the homecoming, everyone is at once full of expectation and fear. No one speaks of it but we all share the apprehension of the next phase of this our collective journey. His mother is much better, his daughter is arranging to spend nights at the house and the McMillan people, GP and pharmacist are all briefed. We are as ready as we can be – for what? I am impressed by his mother's faith, that whatever comes – she will deal with it, his daughter too, is adamant that all will be managed, and my daughter is also calm and committed to making this homecoming a happy one.

CHAPTER TEN

Now things have changed, my son is at home with his mother, she assumes the responsibility that so far I have felt it right to carry. In so doing I have kept my son close to me. Somehow I am relieved and unsettled at once, I am not sure what my role is to be. What I do know is that my son's mother loves her boy without reserve and wants to hold him close in these last days. Although it is many years since we parted, I feel very proud of her, for she is far from fit herself. I believe that she does not know how hard the next week(s) are going to be, so I must be vigilant. She may be loath to share her burden, at least with me. I know that daughter and granddaughter will find time to pitch in and help. Sharing grief is hard, for even in this, we are sometimes selfish. I question my past and my part in the shaping of my son, now a dying drug addict. I keep on asking what if? Why didn't I intervene and face what was staring me in the face? What if his mother and I had held it together and not divorced? So many what ifs!

I go to my home, the fifty or so miles don't seem to matter a jot, there's hope that our son will have a little of life to enjoy, I am just a little confused as to what my role will be. I don't want to impose on his mother nor do I want to be absent from his company. For the first time in all these weeks I share these thoughts with my wife. She listens quietly, she is careful and gentle in her responses, I can hear the eggshells crack under her feet. It is decided that I shall visit each day, though I shall be careful not to step on the toes of his mother. No need to rush out first thing, perhaps get down to him and spend the middle of the day together. If the boy is up to it we can go out for lunch, perhaps a beer together.

My first visit to the house rather than the hospice is bewildering; I don't quite know how I'm expected to behave. I am now a visitor into my ex-wife's home, the house is small and neat, it has recovered from the chaos of our boy's last occupation when everything went so horribly wrong. There is an air of make believe that this time the boy will be better, at least in control. But I know he is not better, each day, each hour, he is being devoured by this monstrous disease.

The spring weather is wonderful, it makes the morning drive very pleasant, I now no longer necessarily take the quickest or shortest route; eventually I develop a routine. I find that at first I cannot help but rush to be with my boy and on some occasions arrive embarrassingly early. Sometimes the household is asleep so I creep around outside or go away and take coffee in the local town.

I always buy a newspaper so that when I sit in the little house made smaller by my son's downstairs quarters, I can perch on the chair and bury my head in the current affairs of the day and remain there; hidden but close to my boy.

Sometimes his daughter has spent the night, so the place is even more crowded, there are duvets and ashtrays, snack trays and all manner of domestic detritus that I find slightly uncomfortable. I strive constantly not to show my discomfort and I am always happy to run errands to the shops or pharmacy or whatever, making myself useful as a member of the team.

When my daughter gets away from work I propose we all go out to lunch, his mother declines, so his sister, my boy and me, we go off to a pub in the country a mile or two away. My boy is dressed in a tracksuit, a baseball cap with trainers on his feet. Apart from his unusual mode of dress he looks appalling and he is able to shuffle about fifty yards max. So where ever we go I have to park very close to the entrance, which on occasions drew some unsympathetic responses from 'Joe Public'. I ignore the stares and help my boy, I see the stares of disapproval melt away as he emerges from my car, they look away and we shuffle to whatever place we need to go.

Sometimes we are just the two of us, sometimes three, his mother never comes. When his daughter is with us; the elder one, we seldom see the younger, they always sit close and touch each other a lot, their affection and love for each other is wonderful. This, his first born child, who I do not really know, continues to be steadfast and true to her father. My daughter too, is the same; holding up her brother and her father with courage and kindness. These two young women are entirely without self consciousness, they have an innocent relationship with my son, unadorned by mistakes and guilt, they know only their unconditional love and affection for my boy. Why am I surprised? Maybe it's because I have been such a lousy father.

At these lunch hours my boy still eats ravenously, sometimes his table manners in these public places are embarrassing, so I try to punctuate the meal with snippets of interrogative conversation in the hope that he will look up from his troughing and perhaps pause for a second or two. He seldom responds. When either of the young women is present they ignore my interventions and politely tell me to keep my counsel.

I coach myself between visits to be ready for catastrophic change, to be aware of his state. It is thee drugs and sedatives that make his life bearable, but I must watch, be vigilant and care for each moment with him, come what may.

On other days we go out together just the two of us. He likes to escape from the house, he wants to be "out".

His mother understands and shoos us out into the spring sunshine. On this day we drive aimlessly through the area; I meander through the byways of my earlier years reminiscing about when we moved here all those years ago. We drive past the factory where my boy was offered a management apprenticeship, I wonder how different things would be had he'd accepted. I tease him about all the advice he scorned. He listens intently, and I feel suddenly guilty that I am somehow chastising him again. He smiles ruefully but says nothing.

Frequently he is quiet, he listens to my endless and aimless chatter. I am trying to fill time, to tell him through this constant, what I hope is good humoured banter, repetitively, and probably boringly that I love him. Not in so many words, but by trying to care for each minute we are together and sharing each other. I am desperate that we shall part as loving friends. My shame and wretchedness about my part in what has come to pass is a bed of thorns. Of all my ambitions in an ambitious life, I have not known such a powerful drive. So as I embellish each minute with my constant chat, I am aware of his silence. My pauses are pregnant, and I am absurdly delighted when he makes the most mundane reply. Sometimes he chuckles and when he does, I am thrilled – we are enjoying ourselves.

When he does talk, it is about his friends I do not know, often about friends who I ought to admire, friends who have made the grade. The message is clear; he is telling me that despite the calamitous drug issue he has had an eventful and often fun filled life. He has regrets but neither of us dwells on those and instead we look back to happy times. We talk about things that are outside of a normal father son parenthesis, we confess to each other some of our worst boyish pranks, avoiding I suppose the most carnal. We are striving to be pals - chums - mates and the great joy is that it is not too late.

These conversations are sometimes relaxed; at least for me. I wonder how he sees them, my boy? As we count the minutes passing, knowing at any moment that the monster within will strike and devour him. He tells me he would like to come to my home, he has never been there, I immediately respond with an idea that has been germinating within me for some time, "Next Sunday," I say, "we'll have a Sunday lunch," I almost blurt out 'a Sunday lunch to remember!' But I check myself in the nick of time.

"Can I bring the girls?" he asks.

"Of Course," I reply.

I look forward and pray we all can make it to the feast.

My discipline about avoiding talking about the future is becoming addled; I find my mind is discovering it increasingly difficult to live in the past. I have now reminisced for weeks and apart from mentioning very short term issues such as appointments and what time I'm going to visit, the future has ceased to exist. However, secretly I count the hours, much as I imagine does my son, watching and waiting for his life to ebb away. Waiting, our nerves on edge, waiting for the monster to strike as it surely will, it might be minutes, hours but I know it will be soon.

He has been home a week, and today the sun shines once more, and the two of us set out to lunch, we drive through the may strewn hedgerows out to our favourite pub. It is a beautiful day. I am watchful that I don't say that it is a beautiful day, I am fearful that this will beg the question – how many more days do we have? There are a few people in the pub, and we settle, my boy with his cider and me with a pint of beer. It is hard for him to walk at all, I notice that now twenty five yards is about all he can manage. He coughs and I see him wince.

I wince in sympathy, I am afraid. We order, and he eats as usual, like a starving animal. My fear recedes.

After lunch I bring the car round and load him in and

set out for home, but just as we are leaving the pub car park he asks me to stop.

"Can I walk by the canal, Dad?"

We stop, it is a very difficult spot, right on a zed bend crossing the canal, but I stop and reverse to the start of the footpath. I help him from the car, I tell him to stay put, and I reverse some more to the pub car park some fifty yards distant. I park and rush to his side. We walk down to the canal, I am letting him lean on me and we shuffle a few yards at a time, we walk under the road bridge and settle on a ledge alongside the canal and overlooking a narrow- boat yard.

It is a delightful day, as beautiful a day as you will ever find in England. The warm late April sun shines on us, the willows weep sweetly, the daffodils peek brightly from the embankment, and the narrow-boats let their bright paint reflect from the canal's green opaque waters. We sit in this idyllic place and he lights a cigarette. I resist a huff.

"It must be lovely to live in a narrow-boat on the canal." He says.

"Looks lovely now," I respond, "but not so good on a cold wet winter's day."

He chuckles, "That's the difference between us, you always think ahead. I would have liked to live on a narrow-boat, it would have been great."

"Well you certainly lived in some curious places," and we chat about his eccentric past before he moved in with his mum.

We both laugh, and then we sit there for a minute or two, savouring the moment.

It's time to take him home, and as we shuffle back to the road, I notice how weak he has become. His breath is short, his foot step tiny, his breath laboured, his eyes stare at the path below his feet, he leans back into me, and I hold him as gently as I can, because I know if I hold him tight he will hurt.

He is tired, but we are both happy in the knowledge that this hour or so has been for us a time of worth, a time when we were alone; the only two on our lonely planet; both of us revelling in the past and desperately trying not to think of the future. I feel him next to me as we shamble towards the road; he is a bag of bones, my son disassembling before my very eyes.

We get home and plan the weekend, my boy will be taken to his sister's home tomorrow, his daughter will also come and then they will all come to my home on Sunday and I will cook a feast. He has never visited my present home, and he has only met my lovely wife on a few recent occasions when he was always in his sick bed. He tells me what a 'nice lady' she is and how he's looking forward to the visit.

For my part I am furiously planning a feast to end all feasts, I will cook the finest Sunday Roast there's ever been, I will because this will be my gift to him, it is the best way I can express my love. On the edge of my cooking ambition is the lurking fear that Sunday will be too late and he will have ceased to eat. I pray fervently for another two days at least when he will eat, for I have seen on that short walk on the canal bank that time is very short.

I bid him and everyone a farewell, he lays down and sleeps. We whisper while he sleeps, "How's he doing? Does he seem comfortable? Do you think we should let his pals take him out tonight?" His mother and I worry, his sister tells us to mind our business and let my boy make his own decisions whilst he can. As ever she is so much wiser than us parents. I resist the urge to ask everyone to be careful, watch this, watch that; it is too late for that. "See you on Sunday," I say, as I swagger out of the little house, my swagger is all pretend.

CHAPTER ELEVEN

It is Saturday I am obsessed with creating tomorrow's lunch, the guest list is my wife, my daughter and her partner, my granddaughter, and my son. It is not unusual in the sense that I have been preoccupied with food and eating for most of my life, and now it is my wont to cook and break bread as a symbol of my caring for those I love.

Today and tomorrow though is different, I know in my heart of hearts that this meal will literally be my son's last, certainly with me in my home. It is my last chance to give him something that is unique and will give him a sensual as well as a spiritual gift, a tangible expression of my love, and an apology for what might have been.

For my wife who has only met my son a few times in the hospital, it must be an anxious time, but I confess that I take her for granted. Through all these dreadful weeks she has been a patient and generous bystander who has respected my grief and nurtured me in my pain, and all of this she has suffered without a word of disagreement or angst. She watches me now as I dash about like a demented TV cook and suffers her fool gladly.

I plot the unfolding adventure of my son's journey to his sister's together with the older grandchild. I have learned in these awful weeks the effectiveness of mobile communications, I have bought gizmos of varying complexity that keep me open and in touch with my son and his carers at all times. I have managed to become a nuisance on an epic scale. Today I transfer my assault to butchers and grocers as my menu for the feast takes shape. As always; no matter who the expected guests, my wife cleans and hoovers while I chop, and season, mix and taste, chill and flavour. The day passes in a flurry of nervous expectation, we are exhausted by the day's end, we must now sleep if we can, and await the arrival of my boy.

A bright day dawns, I am already awake watching another day inch its way into being, first light and then the brash sun urging me to get out of bed. It is still early, my wife slumbers on as I creep out of bed, and wonder about checking my watch and arguing with myself whether it is or is not too early to check on my son's welfare. It is only seven o clock, too early I am sure, I imagine him sleeping; hoping that his strength this day is going to be enough to enjoy the feast. I am nervous, about whether he will be well, about how his daughter will respond, about the stress on my wife, and not least about the lunch; The roasting of the luscious bird, the stuffing, the pigs in their blankets, and the roast potatoes to name but a few of the details.

It is Sunday and I pause to think about what Sunday used to be, it meant church and village routine, now I know my faith is rattled even defeated utterly. All the old intellectual arguments come back; the reasons not to believe despite my christian upbringing. I see my son's struggle and suffering as a cold reminder of the realities of existence, and his dismissal of the hereafter as a brave statement of the obvious. Should I feel glad that when he dies he has no fear of the afterlife, or should I be afraid that he's exposing his immortal coil to eternal damnation?

I hear the stirring from the bedroom and love in the shape of my wife lights the room and all the arguments retreat in confusion.

A kitchen drama is at hand, and the next hours are gobbled up preparing the feast. I learn by telephone that all is well at my daughter's home and the party sets out on schedule, my timings are adjusted in the kitchen with the precision of a space mission. The tension builds; it cannot be greater if a head of state were our guest. My nerves are on edge, beyond the mere issues of the food: How will my boy react? And my granddaughter how will she be? Neither of them have any idea how I live and I am worried that they will see and perceive a standard of living they have not shared because of our separate developments. I am being absurd, I am afraid they will think that I have deserted them and gone on to live a life that has been so much more comfortable than theirs. As the years have passed, I reflect in my nervous dithering in the kitchen, I have seen less and less of them, partly through my boy's avoidance of me, but largely because I chose to give up and avert my eyes from what has been an inconvenience. If they rail against me, and call me the names I deserve, how will I react, I am afraid of the retribution. My hands shake as I prepare my offering. I pray to I know not who, that the next hours go well, that we are kind to each other, that we enjoy this communion. I know I can rely on my daughter and my wife to smooth the way, I know that my boy and I have come a long way together in these past weeks, I know my granddaughter is a fine and gutsy girl, but I remain afraid.

I don't know who the patron saint of cooking is, but whoever it is, he guards me well and everything in the kitchen is going to plan, the smells are divine, the dishes are all coming together, everything is in order, all we need now is the guests to appear on time, and indeed as I look through the kitchen window I see them arrive. We wait as the party comes up in the lift, and they are here. He stands in the doorway, grey and emaciated his untidy beard unable to hide his sunken cheeks. His eyes are still alight, he smiles, I put my arms out to welcome him, "Come in, come in." I greet them all with exaggerated bonhomie, "go through, go through," we're all hugging, and I see my son and his daughter taking in the view of my middle class living. Drinks are dispensed, g and tees from my wife and me, cider for my boy, a beer for my daughter's partner, and coke for granddaughter and daughter.

"Lovely flat," says my boy. "Can I have a look round?"

He and his daughter are taken on a tour of the place by my wife. My daughter and I whisper about the night that has passed. All went well and my nerves settle as the first part of the pattern I seek, falls into place.

He returns with his daughter gently helping him and my wife bringing up the rear. "Lovely place, Dad, really nice," he says, there is no malice in his voice, he is glad for me.

My granddaughter too, proclaims her delight, she is starry eyed as if in a toy shop, she takes in the furniture, the curtains and the pictures. I imagine I see a flicker of regret at what she's missed, but there is no ill feeling.

It is not long before my son and his daughter seek permission to have a cigarette, so they go together, a conspiracy of smokers, onto the balcony and satisfy their addiction. I say nothing, I dare not as my daughter watches, ready to pounce, if I so much as witter one word about my aversion to tobacco.

When they have finished their infusion of nicotine, I can no longer resist a barbed dart and despite myself blurt out; "When you've not had a cigarette for four weeks, my dear, we'll see a lot more of you."

My granddaughter smiles an indulgent smile, "I will give up, I promise."

"Good girl," I reply anxious to move on, "Come on, it's time for lunch. Hungry everybody?"

"Starving, Dad," says my boy; my heart sings, my offering will be worthwhile.

If a casual observer looked at us now, he would see nothing unusual. A family at Sunday lunch, good humour, affection, warmth and kindness. For me it is impossible to escape the reference to the last supper, except there sits at the head of the table, no saint, but my boy, now so wasted and clutching so desperately to life. He appears to be enjoying the moment; yet he must be in an agony of uncertainty. I am astonished and euphoric at how he is engaged, eating with gusto, and in happy conversation with his sister and daughter who flank him. This moment is more than I could have asked for, it is a time I will forever cherish.

There are oohs and ahs as the dessert is presented, my wife's offering, it is delicious and vanishes in a trice. And soon, so soon lunch is over, and we break away from the table and the boy and his daughter make another sortie to the balcony for their inevitable cigarette.

Later we sit and chat, and I notice the absence of my son, and then I see the toes of his shoes protrude from the top of the settee; he is sound asleep. He sleeps for an hour or more and when he awakes, despite the offer of tea, it is time that he should go.

"Thanks Dad," he says, "It's been great, really enjoyed it."

"Me too," says my granddaughter, "thank you both very much." She is polite but genuine, she kisses my cheek and hugs my wife.

My boy does likewise; he hugs me and touched my neck with his gargantuan fingers, I sense his affection, I try not to squeeze him as I bid him farewell. "I will see you tomorrow."

"Don't bother, tomorrow, Dad," he says, "I'll be fine, have a rest." And he's off shuffling into the lift. His sister and daughter escorting his frail frame, the afternoon is over. We watch from the kitchen as they drive away. My wife says nothing, she holds me and I weep. My tears are tears of joy and grief, we have together, all of us, delivered an hour or two of joy, we have collectively created a precious circle of love that will last forever.

CHAPTER TWELVE

Through sundry phone calls I learn all is well, my boy has slept well but is exhausted. I am urged to stay at home and rest.

I have to confess to feeling very, very tired. I am weary through to my bones, my heart aches with the constant pain of grief, and my mind aches with the constant worry of "what's next?" It's a question that never recedes, there is no peace, as time flies and my son's enemy within lies in wait for the last push.

All through these dark days I have lived in such a small world, everything except those things involved in the drama of my boy's existence have ceased to exist. It is easy to become obsessed with my own struggle and forget those others who are equally or even more tortured.

His mother who is so quiet, sometimes she seems so detached, so stoic, it is easy to assume she cares less, but I know this is not true. Her mobility is a problem and the stress of looking after our son at her home has been immense. Inevitably I have mused about those years past when our marriage broke down, when the young woman so full of adventure and fun changed into someone shy and withdrawn. She was the one who, alone, held her children close, she was the one who struggled with their teenage tantrums and woes, she was the one who saw our boy every day sink slowly but surely into the abyss of his addiction. Now she weeps alone, her strength all but sapped by the years of her solace. Part of me weeps for her, for today like every day I remember so well that wail of pain, when she learned of her boy's demise, it was terrible; it was the cry of all mothers for all the lost sons, it echoes in my soul.

Then there are his children, my grandchildren. I hardly know them; over the years since their birth I have never been close. They were born to my son's girlfriend, someone I had never met at the time of the first birth. At the time I was disappointed and vexed to think a son of mine would get a girl pregnant without even the pretext of a long term commitment between them. Maybe there was such a commitment, but there were no warnings of their relationship, its foundation, or of any planned future. I remember learning from my estranged wife that my son had made some girl pregnant, the girl whoever she was, anonymous and suddenly a de facto member of our dysfunctional family. I accepted the news with undisguised displeasure; the events were, in my view were another indicator of my son's departure from my idea of normality or acceptable behaviour. That phase in our lives set the tone for the years ahead, the alienation of my son through me growing ever more aloof and arrogantly distant.

So what do they think of me now, my grandchildren? It's hard to say, I am more worldly, older by far, more confident, more comfortably off. If I were them, I would dislike me and I can easily see why. In all my grief and pain I still find it hard to connect, the absence has been too deliberate; I have denied them for too long.

They are innocent, like kittens, they curl up beside me looking for warmth but I am incapable of giving them what they want. I see courage and fearlessness in the older and confusion in the younger, and I see devotion in them both toward their father. When he goes, where will they seek their futures where will they anchor their hope? Who will be their mentor? I have no answer.

I see in the older child strength of character, someone who can make a good life for herself, she has guts and she'll need them if she is to escape from the environment that I have only glimpsed. For the younger sister I see a kind but shallower young woman, content with her lot, and a naivety that leaves her so vulnerable. I gather that everyone at their home smokes, no one except her grandmother is in gainful employment, and that their maternal grandfather also died from lung cancer, and yet they continue to smoke. I suspect that their mother, like my son, has been addicted to drugs other than tobacco.

My escape route from my own grandfatherly responsibilities is that I will promise to keep in contact if, and only if, my granddaughters give up smoking. Part of me wishes fervently that they give up their addiction, part of me hopes they stay out of my life. I am ashamed; I am a coward who is not prepared to pay my son's debt. I do not have the strength to nurture what I know that he wants me to nurture, as I failed him in life, I know I will fail him again after he is gone. My resolve now is weak, only the grandchildren can strengthen me, it is a two way street, where I do not want to walk.

There is a boy, he is not of my son's blood, but he is a half brother to the girls, I have only met him once when he was very small. Despite this boy having a living father he has been devoted to my boy and calls him 'Dad'. Since my boy has lived in penury feeding his drug habit, it seems astonishing to me that he should adopt in day to day terms this unrelated boy, and to love him. That is clearly the case. Latterly my boy has included this unknown lad in all his expressed desires to leave legacies from his pathetically small estate.

Since the day I first understood, I have been sustained by two women, my new wife and my daughter, my boy's sister. My wife has given me safe harbour and a tranquil haven of support. She has watched my obsession grow and eased my agony. She has been silent when silence has been my balm, she has been my counsellor when I have been in danger of losing my senses, she has been my nurse when I have felt so exhausted and down. She has been my angel of mercy, she has loved me selflessly.

My daughter is in the middle of this unfolding tragedy. She is a young and attractive woman, she has spirit and resilience, she shares her brother's sometimes outrageous sense of humour. She lives with her partner who through all this harrowing time has, I fancy, been as supportive to my daughter as my wife has been to me. She is two years younger than her brother. We are close; she nursed me through the loss of my second wife who died so suddenly and traumatically. I believe she understands me, that she is a chip off the old block and I love her dearly and with great affection. She has been the bridge between her mother and me. Through all the years or our irregular meetings there was never a time we did not discuss her mother and her brother. He was in those days perceived by us as the zany off the wall member of the family who was beyond our humdrum existence. We had discussed many times our views that my boy was on drugs, but she always reassured me that maybe he smoked a bit of pot, but that was it. I chose to take comfort from her words; my blind eye was intensely focused on what I wanted to see.

We have reprised these conversations many times over the last month or so; we bob and weave through our dialogue knowing it's too late now to change a thing. Despite my unsureness of what we really believed, she has been my closest kindred spirit; her devotion to her brother has been without reserve. She has spent nights with him and travelled so many hours after hard days at work. She is exhausted and I see the wear on her persona, she looks older now than when we first met at the hospital just eight weeks ago. It seems an age has passed. It is impossible for me to love my daughter more than I already do, apart from the fact that love is absolute – you do or you don't – but now I am proud of her. She is generous and kind, strong and sensitive, courageous and funny, beautiful and loving – what a lucky man I am.

Despite the tragedy of my boy's life, there shines through a gentle loving man who adores his children. Who, despite his indecent existence, is the everyday essence of decency; he is kind, gentle, amusing, courageous and loving. Although his adult life has passed in a fog of drug induced dizziness, and he has missed many things that I hold to be of value, he has held on to love. I cannot imagine the horrors of his past, the desperation of feeding his insatiable habit, the loneliness of being locked out by his shame and the need to hide away from those he loves, and the physical torments of deprivation and chaotic lifestyle. The many cold lonely nights and all the misery and emptiness of being an outcast should have bred bitterness, but I see no signs of it.

I must not guild the lily, he fell because of weakness and once he succumbed he has been, and is, lost. He still is unable to make the daughters he loves so much, give up the weed, in the full and ghastly knowledge of the consequences. His addictions have blanked out his sense of responsibility toward his mother who has looked after him these last eight years and he has been unable or unwilling to spare us all the devastation that is with us now.

Are we to forgive him? Yes, we do, because he loves us and we love him. Our love, his and ours, unconditional. This love burdens us and holds us up, it drains us and sustains us, it holds us together and it will torture us when we part.

CHAPTER THIRTEEN

I keep in touch as always, and my boy seems to have got home to his mothers with minimal discomfort. I am still basking in the comfort of how well the day went yesterday – it really was a delightful get together and both my wife and I are so pleased that he came to visit and share our hospitality. It went so well I think that he has many more days left, though part of me casts doubt over my optimism. I spend the day doing the chores that have been left unattended all this week, as close to good humour and contentment as I have been for weeks.

In my afternoon call to his mother she tells me he remains well, though tired, he did not eat his lunch she says, "You fed him too well yesterday". She says this casually, I can almost hear her smile over the telephone, she is being kind to me.

He did not eat, he did not eat! The hammer hits me, my mouth runs dry, my heart hammers, my breath is short – he did not eat!

My hubris dies in a flash, my wife as sensitive as ever sees my shoulders slump my gait stiffen. I reply blandly to his mother, I mutter my thanks for her compliment, but I know beyond certainty that my boy is moving quickly toward his end.

I discuss what I have learned with my wife. "It is" I say, "the beginning of the last lap, once his appetite goes all his other functions will begin to disassemble and he will die soon, very soon." My wife asks how I know. I know, sadly I know beyond doubt.

I wait for my daughter to come home from work and I ring her and tell her the news. She understands immediately, I hear her hold back her tears. As ever she dashes into action and says she'll dash down to be at his side.

I am spent, I am worried and I am confused as to what it is that I should do next. I am clear that my boy's loss of appetite is the first domino to fall, before his final curtain, but I am not clear how quickly the other functions will collapse. I am tempted to ring the hospice but I am loath to burden them when the answer will probably be "It's hard to say and no two cases are the same". His mother did not report any other symptoms, so I prowl the house, ruminating on what will happen next. I shall get down there early tomorrow and see how things are going – perhaps he will recover a bit and come out with me as usual, perhaps his Mum was right, I did overdo the feast a bit.

I sleep fitfully, my dreams are unpleasant, full of death and darkness, full of tears and sadness, in my waking I begin to think about what I shall say when he is gone.

It is dawn, on a May morning, the sun shines through the bedroom blinds casting a luminous hue through our too large bedroom. My wife sleeps beside me, her soft snore a confirmation of our comfort together. I listen to her and see what peace there is in her almost silent purring. I am awake and waiting, I am like a tiger waiting to spring upon the events of the day whatever they turn out to be, I lie there watching the light grow stronger, waiting, waiting and then the peace is shattered – the telephone rings and alarms the day, I leap up and my worst fears are confirmed. There are tears and devastation on the end of the phone; my boy has deteriorated so quickly over night, he is in agony he seems to be entirely irrational and is hard to restrain.

The fifty miles are covered at a speed not countenanced by the law; I arrive well before eight a.m. to find a shambles, a bedlam, a storm of chaos. My boy is hardly recognisable, I am not sure he sees me at all. It is as if the devil is abroad and in him and through him, if it were not my boy I would be very frightened. His dignity has been wrenched away, before my eyes and the eyes of his mother daughter and Aunt is the wreckage of a human being ravaged by this monstrous cancer and all the other complications caused by his addiction, it is clear to me that he is deranged, deranged by pain, or the onset of calcium flooding, or the failure of his organs. His mother has been by his side since the beginning of this catastrophic downturn and has ministered to him. She looks shattered, next to her boy she does not weep; I see her willing him to come back to her, not to leave her like this, wild and tortured, without hope.

There is no hope, we are all of us faced with a black hole of despair. My boy's suffering is beyond imagination and there are no drugs that seem to assuage the ravaging pain and confusion. I ring the hospice and as always they listen to what I have to say, it is barely eight o clock. No one can take the decisions yet but they say "Hold on." and they will get back to me, and of course they do. They ask if I can bring him in my car, I doubt that I can; things are too chaotic. They can receive him at ten o clock and an ambulance will be arranged.

So we wait in the terrible confusion, none of us is able to do anything to assuage my boy's agony; he is at least for the moment – nobody we know. He is consumed by this terrible alien within him, his mind and body are disassembling before our collective eyes.

I see the pain in his mother; she is bewildered, exhausted and afraid. She is afraid not of what is happening, but because she knows the reaper has come to collect in the meanest cruellest way possible. It is tearing the life out of him ounce by ounce, second by second. The wait for the ambulance drags on, each moment punctuated by the clatter of my boy's spilling things, dropping things, moaning and cursing.

We try but we cannot comfort him, he does not recognise us from moment to moment, and when he does, we are in turn repulsed and then urged to help. Every attempt to hold him, or even to speak to him are met with irrational responses without any sequence or order. Chaos, evil chaos stalks the little house and we do our best to fight and hold firm with what gentleness we can muster in the face of this monster – 'cancer' is too kind a word to describe it.

At last the ambulance arrives, I assure my boy we are taking him back to where he will have his pain eased, his confusion calmed; to where he will be cared for with a love that he already knows. He hears me and he does not resist.

The ambulance crew is a man and a woman, the woman firmly in charge. We ease my boy into his wheelchair and he is shunted unceremoniously into the ambulance. The crew do not talk to my boy; they do not try to reassure him. I take an instant dislike to them because I do not perceive any sympathy from them. But at least they are efficient.

I race the ambulance to the hospice, I arrive before them and dash to reception and babble to the unflappable volunteer receptionist my plight. She asks me to sit, I find this impossible and pace about in reception. I peep cautiously into the chapel or contemplation room but I cannot bring myself to go in. Time ticks on interminably. I have seen the ambulance arrive what seems like hours ago, I debate whether to harass the receptionist again but decide against it.

Eventually, some twenty minutes after my arrival I am invited to go through. I almost sprint down the corridors I know so well, and in the midst of this short journey I realise that I don't know where they have taken him. I plough on anyway and go to the room he had previously occupied and I am relieved to see him perched half seated half lying in his comfortable bed.

The lady doctor attending him leaves as I arrive; she says nothing apart from a cursory greeting, I barely see her and walk immediately to my boy. Our old friend the nurse who has been so good to him, and us, is attending him, she is securing a subcutaneous drip into his pathetic wizened arm. My boy sees me and I hear him say urgently, "Does he understand the situation?" He turns again to the nurse and says again, "Does Dad understand the situation?"

"Yes," she replies, "he understands the situation."

I am at his side I take his hand in mine, and he looks into my eyes. Yes, I understand the situation, his eyes slowly close and he lapses into unconsciousness.

I am terrified, what did I see? Was it fear? Is my boy alone in his drug induced blackness, alone with his fear, or in panic of dying, of leaving unsaid all the things he wanted to say? My terror rips at my heart, for I know now; I will never speak to him again. I can do nothing except stay close to him and will him to know I love him.

I look up at the nurse as she tidies up. "Last lap?" I say. Her eyes move imperceptibly, 'last lap' it is. The nurse leaves and I cry my dry tears for there is little left.

My boy seems comfortable, his breathing is steady, I hold his hand until my shoulder aches from my awkward posture. I must ring home and tell them he is settled. I must also tell everyone who is close to him, that his time has almost come, so come and visit if you want, come and bid your farewells.

It is a long slow day, my son lies there, and he seems to be at peace. This in itself is respite, and I find myself wondering if I want his end to come. Is there an angel of mercy?

I hope that in his sleep and as his life slips away that the peace I imagine is real. There is part of me that nags away that this cannot be, I am haunted by his urgent last words; "Does he understand the situation?" I do not; I grieve for him locked in a dark peace or is it a nightmare, his road to nemesis.

The day passes, my daughter and his daughter come, each in their beauty clothed in compassion and haunted by grief. They are so lovely, and I know my boy loves them, or loved them? We embrace and I try to mutter words of comfort. "At peace," I say, "His suffering will soon be over" and other platitudes. I seek to shield them from my fears, I find comfort in their tears, the turbulence of my soul is made quiet by their devotion. There is something of the team about us, I can feel their affection and their will to support me, it is a wonderful thing that binds us, I hope my boy can feel it too.

His mother comes, and others too, I am weary, and I become impatient. There is something prurient about sitting round his bed; waiting and watching, waiting and watching for it all to come to an end.

His sister and my daughter will stay the night, my day has come to an exhausting end and I journey home. Tomorrow I will stay over at the hospice and my boy will die. I do not understand how I know this; but I do.

CHAPTER FOURTEEN

Home is indeed my refuge; I tell my wife what I know beyond all certainty. As ever she listens quietly and pats my hand and gently kisses me. "There, there" she says, "it will soon be over." Her words are like gentle rain on parched and tired earth. Yes it will soon be over, and yet I am loath to let him go.

The evening passes slowly, I talk to my daughter on watch at the hospice, we whisper on the phone like guilty lovers sharing a secret. "No change," I mutter after each call.

And so to bed; and a restless night of dreams, and endless minutes of solitude. I dream dreams that my son is dreaming, as he marches toward black eternity. I wake suddenly and weep that he may be afraid, and I hear time and again his cry "Does he know the situation?" I see the anxiety and the fright, or is it terror, in his eyes. I reach out to him but wake sweating restrained by the blankets. I repeat the cycle many times, each time the horror remains the same.

It is dawn and I am awake, my body is made of lead. I am so tired I can barely breathe; the exhaustion is like a thousand weights that tether me to my bed. I hear the gentle purr of my wife beside me and I fight the desire to hold her and love her. The lead weights win, and it is not long before she wakes. Her hands find me and stroke my battered brow, tears roll down my face; welcome to another day.

The shower helps wash away the scars of the night, I give myself a pep talk, 'I must be strong, one last effort, one more heave, one more day.' I am urged not to rush, to take my time, but my son has very little time, I want to share what is left.

The morning calls are comforting, there is no change, he sleeps quietly on. "Very peaceful." My daughter tells me, and I mutter or feign my relief, I keep my secret about the 'situation.'

I pack my overnight bag, I hug my wife and make my way along those fifty or so miles that is my road to Calvary, my car hurtles its way on automatic pilot, my mind is numbly neutral. There is a traffic jam. I curse the idiot responsible although I have no idea who it is, or indeed what the cause is at all, has someone died? The jam clears and my chariot takes off on automatic pilot once more. I arrive at the hospice and my daughter is waiting for me so she can get off to work, my son's daughter has already gone off to school.

"See you tonight," she says.

"See you tonight," I reply.

"God, Dad you don't look well."

"Not so good yourself."

We chuckle hug, and off she goes my brave girl, who I love so much, who has shown me her true lovely grown up self. She is beautiful to look at, beautiful to know; maybe I haven't been such a lousy father after all.

I kiss my son's damp brow; I feel his pulse which is steady but weak. I sit and get used to being with him, because that is all I can do – be with him. Does he know I'm here? These constant impossible questions are wearing me down. I try not to think at all – it is impossible.

The nurses are astonishing, they come and go, they keep my son clean and comfortable, but more than that they talk to him and me as if we are all in the conversation. They smile, they pat him with affection and they care for this part of his life as they have done all along. They are sublimely kind; once more I am humbled to a point of weeping. I feel embarrassed; I excuse myself and go out to get a newspaper. Once outside I become aware of my crassness and then drive to the paper shop with dangerous speed, I am irrational and I know it. I rush back with the irrationality telling me that he will be gone by the time I return. I am away only ten minutes, I rush to his room; nothing has changed. I sit breathless, beginning to wonder about my certainty about his time.

There then begins a stream of visitors, at first I welcome them, but soon I find it difficult to make conversation.. They sit around my son's bed and mutter banalities. I am getting impatient, "Go away," I want to tell them, "go away, piss off, leave us alone." I don't say it, but I think it in spades. I am reminded of my boy when the chaplain came to visit, I know what he felt, "Bugger off and let me die with those I choose." That's what he meant and I understand.

His mother comes, his aunt, his ex-partner the mother of his children, his children, the boy who was not his blood son but his adopted one, they sit around his bed like so many Indians in a tepee. Despite their claims on him, I cannot surrender my paternal role, at least as I see it. I find myself watching each person in turn. I find them prurient, gawping at a dying man, and inept, the conversation becomes unbearable. I mutter there are too many people in the room and I leave and sit in the little coffee room alone. I cannot wait for them to leave so I can have my son back. Alone in the coffee room I know that I am being completely unreasonable, mean minded, selfish, but still I want them all to go. Well not all, I want his mother to stay. I want her to be at his parting, though I know she will not be there. She is battered and bruised and beaten, she is as vulnerable as it is possible to be. I do not understand how she has borne the decline of our boy over the years, has rebuffed my queries and worries, defending him even when he was killing himself. I do not want her to suffer any more; there has been enough of it.

Eventually everyone departs and I am glad.

Evening is here, the promiscuous ducks are settling on the duck pond, I wait for the A team, my daughter who is coming from work and my granddaughter who is coming to share the vigil after her day at College.

My daughter comes first, she hugs me, she looks at her brother, speaks to him as though he were aware of us.

"Any change?"

"No change, but I feel it won't be long." I take her hand and we settle at my boy's bedside. It is quiet there is not much to say.

My granddaughter comes; we go through the same ritual.

It is nine o'clock, we, the three of us, have been variously sitting, mooching, making tea, chatting quietly, there is no impatience; time is standing as still as it can. We are all watching and waiting, for the ripples on the pool of his life to stop. We tend him gently, swab his lips, mop his brow, and whisper "there there, good boy," or "dad, or his name." We wait; our hearts beating loudly in our breasts, our own breath tentative as we watch the hypnotic rise and fall of his breathing. We all breathe in subconscious unison.

The nurses come and go; their superhuman good humour carries them brusquely about their business. They know what is unfolding and yet they are sympathetic but uncannily cheerful. Their cheerfulness lifts us, not much but enough to be patient, to know that what is unfolding is not a trial of unique tragedy, but an everyday event; something that has to be lived with. Their attention to the patient is as meticulous as ever, they talk to the dying boy with a sweet matter of factness that shows they care for this moment as they have cared for every other, they confirm he is alive and that they care. There is no giving up, there is no hopelessness here, there is only care.

I go to make coffee and beside me I see a little lady, about fifty maybe younger. I bid her good evening; she replies in a quiet voice, I hardly hear her. We clatter our tea cups, I try again, I enquire rather clumsily about her circumstances. I hear that she is not a local, she is foreign and as soon as we talk it is as if a damn breaks and she tells me everything.

She is Romanian, her husband is dying, she expects him not to last the night, maybe hours, she has a small child who is there at the back of the room exhausted and bewildered. The Romanian lady asks about my predicament, I reply and tell her that I too, expect my boy to die within hours, she says, "Sorry." And we part.

The girls are tired, and they decide to go to bed, they will sleep in the lovely rooms set aside for relatives. The girls make me promise that if anything should 'happen' I will call them, I reassure them that I will. We hug and off they go, my two super troopers to, I hope, a good rest.

The nurses wheel in a reclining chair for me, and fuss about my boy. They refill the mouth swab, and we chat. The nurse pats me on my arm, I feel her affection and her sweet kindness, and it warms my spirit. I experiment with the comfortable electrically driven chair, it is very comfortable indeed. I must not sleep lest he slips away, I tell him so quietly, I reassure him that I will be there by his side. I mop his brow and check his pulse; he is very damp he is sweating profusely. His breath is shallow but still he clings to life. I tell him a bedtime story, it's not a very good one; it's about a father who lost his son and what could have been. I talk for hours, taking time to moisten his mouth and pat his brow, but sleep creeps up on me. I wake with a start, I hear the nurse walking down the corridor, I panic; my boy is still with me. I go through my nursing routine again; I admonish my weary body for being so weak. I stretch my legs, it is four in the morning, I hear a muffled cry from down the corridor, I wonder about the Romanian lady.

I listen to my boy as he breathes evermore gently, I find myself waiting, almost willing it to be over. It is a tussle between my fears and my hopes. And still relentlessly in the background I hear his last words; 'Does he know the situation?' and the look of alarm in his eye. I pray for his peace, to whom I pray, I am not at all sure. I am asleep once more and wake up once more, and each time it is the same; a start, a panic and the relief to know that my boy's still there. I can care a little more, moisten his lips and mouth and dry his head and shoulders. When I squeeze the swab gently into his mouth I must be careful not to choke him, not to put too much liquid into his airways. I whisper that I am there, in the ridiculous hope that he is aware of my presence. I sit back and the process repeats itself.

It is quite light, I am fully awake, my boy is, as far as I can see, unchanged. I hear the hospice awake, the nurses beginning to start their morning routine; they come in and seem quite spritely after their long night shift. I make a coffee, and soon, it is six forty my daughter and granddaughter emerge in their nightgowns checking on my boy. I report little change and they dart off to shower and get dressed. I sit once more and chat some more, my monologue without much purpose, and then I hear the rhythm change, his breathing becomes irregular.

I hold his hand and call the nurse, "Quick," I say, "fetch the girls, they're dressing. My boy is passing." Despite myself, I cannot help but pray: "The Lord bless you and keep you, may his countenance shine upon you and give you peace."

He dies, it takes a moment or two and the girls rush in, and they catch his last breath. They weep and cry, and hold each other and cling to the nurses who are now with us. The nurses, caring as always tell them to disengage and come to me. I am silent, I do not weep, all is at rest, all is free all is immortal. I hold the girls silently. It is ten past seven in the morning.

The three of us stand there not able to move, a life has passed and his still grey body lies motionless and cold.

"Come," I say, "Don't dwell too long, let's remember him alive and well, with his impish smile." They don't move. I wait a moment, "I must go tell his Mum."

"Can't you phone," says my granddaughter.

"No I can't, I must go, I won't be long."

It is the thirteenth of May, the sun is shining and I emerge into the bright car park, glad to get away, dazed as if I had just completed a great physical encounter. The fight is over; he is gone. The inevitable has come about; he is no more, at least in my time dimension. I muse about my lost faith, my scepticism of a life hereafter, and my boy's stoic view and refusal to seek redemption. It saddens me but I cling to the minimum hope that at least he is now at peace.

It is a short ride to his mother's home, they will just be getting up, so I dawdle through the morning traffic. I make no plan, I rehearse no words, I am numb and sad that whatever I do or say, it will inflict yet more pain. My punch drunk soul is short of compassion, my tank is empty – just one more step and my job at least for the moment will be done.

I ring home and speak to my wife, I tell her as if rehearsing, "he died at ten past seven, he died peacefully." I tell her I am on the way to my boy's mother.

She is more concerned for me, "take time, take care, come home when you can," she tells me she loves me and I am glad, a small light to show me the way.

I arrive at his mother's house, I tap the door and her sister answers the door, she tells me my former wife is dressing and will be down in a moment I wait in the little house that has been restored to its prim and tidy state. As I wait it is hard to believe that only four days ago this place was chaos. I accept a cup of tea. His mother emerges, I put down my teacup and walk to her my arms ahead of me, "He is gone, our boy died this morning at ten past seven."

We hug, she weeps quietly. We disengage, she wipes her eyes. "I want to go to him," she says, " I must go to him now." There is no room for argument. She will travel back to the hospice with her sister I will return as well, not sure any more what I should be doing. I promise to meet her there; back at the hospice.

When I return to my boy's resting place, his other daughter, his former partner are all there sitting around my son's body, all weeping and wailing. I can't bear it, I leave the room as soon as I enter in a brutally quick about turn. My daughter notices and come to my side, I don't want to say anything but she coaxes me into an outburst I immediately regret.

"He's dead, he's gone, why are they all being hysterical round the husk that was his body, bloody gawping, why didn't they all look after him when he was alive?" I pause, "Why didn't I?"

My daughter says nothing, just hugs me and soothes me. His mother arrives and joins the throng around the dead boy. I take my farewells and gather myself to arrange the things that must be arranged. I talk to the staff about death certificates and all the peculiar issues relating to the business of death.

They are very helpful and sensitive, they tell me when to come and collect documents, and they will make appointments for me with the Registrar, then there is my awkward approach about collecting my son's body. They say – no rush take your time, let us know when you've had time to appoint an undertaker.

I drive the long journey home, to the safe harbour of my lovely wife's embrace; there seems no future and no past.

CHAPTER FIFTEEN

I am absorbed by the administration of death and all the paraphernalia that attends the end of life. I take on the responsibility because it is clearly mine, I am the senior member of the clan, he, the subject is my son.

I am confused, not so much about what my boy wanted, in terms of how we mark the end of his life, I am concerned about departing from my own way of life and the assumptions that lie so deeply in my psyche. I have after all buried or cremated a father, mother, and wife and now I must do the same for my boy. But what to do? His rejection of the kindly chaplain seemed so definite, so clear; I feel the imperative to do as he would want. I talk to my daughter and we decide that the way he would want it, would be to go the non religious way.

I acquiesce, but deep, deep down I am uneasy.

First, however it is time to collect death certificates, so two days after my boy's death my wife and I, make an appointment to do so. Once we have collected the medical paperwork from the hospice, we proceed to the registrar. It is strange visiting the hospice that place that cares for life, for now there is, as far as I am concerned, no life left to care for. Now when we visit we are strangers, the carers are fighting new battles with new patients, with the same brusque devotion that we had been used to. The papers are handed over respectfully, by someone I have never met before. There is no familiarity, no connection; there is emptiness, a disappointment that I do not belong here anymore. It is very matter of fact. It hurts.

The Registrar's Office is but a few hundred yards away in the midst of a grandly landscaped set of offices, complete with lake and ancient trees. The offices are vast and modern with glass walls and sculptures and discreet signs, pointing to the offices of a thousand civil servants all no doubt doing worthy things, slaving selflessly for the people of the county. Despite all the signs we find it confusing and we have to ask the way to the Registrar's lair. We arrive I am apprehensive amongst all this formality, it's all so massive and formal, I feel small.

We duly arrive at the Registrar's we are fifteen minutes early, nevertheless we ring the bell and sit and wait in the beautifully furnished reception room. A young man receives us, and tut tuts – "you are early" – He states with some solemnity that we should return at the appointed hour and suggests perhaps we would be more comfortable waiting in the canteen. We retreat as directed into what is a splendid canteen that would do credit to a top class hotel, though I am not able to judge the quality of the food. We wait rather aimlessly and watch the sundry civil servants come and go, I am impatient to be sitting here drinking indifferent coffee just to fill in the twelve minutes to meet the registrar, I have a certainty that the registrar is drinking tea waiting for the appointed hour – what a way to order one's life.

The twelve minutes pass and we present ourselves back at the Registrar's reception and we are asked to sit, but only for the hand of the clock to hit eleven o clock precisely at which point we are ushered into the sterile office where we are greeted by the Registrar. She is middle aged dressed appropriately in a dark lady's suit with a crisp white blouse primly fastened to her throat. She greets us solemnly, shakes our hands and we sit, I hand over the documents from the hospice. The registrar reads them in silence, then she seeks to get my identity, and asks me a lot of questions, about my son's death;

"Was there anyone with him when he died?"

"Yes," I reply.

"Was anyone else present?"

"Yes."

"Who?"

"His sister, his daughter and two nurses from the Hospice."

She seems satisfied. She unsheathes a certificate, types in the details, and then with great ceremony unscrews her fine fountain pen and signs the certificate. She enquires how many copies I require and lets me know the charge per copy, signs several more and delivers the death certificates in a pristine envelope. We are done; the whole process took around six minutes.

We emerge into the cool grey day, I am numb. My wife takes my hand, "and what's next?" she asks.

"Funeral arrangements." Just the two words and we trudge to the car and we make our way to the funeral directors his mother has chosen.

As I enter the funeral Directors I am assailed by a smell that is so vivid, it takes me back sixty years. It is the smell of flowers mixed with the scent of wood, I see in my mind's eye my brother's coffin of sixty years before. His body lay in our front room for three days before he was buried. I was ten then and as I sit here now I am momentarily ten again.

The young lady who receives us strikes a measured balance of welcome and respect, she smiles and her smile, though practised, radiates comfort.

I present the documents and explain where my son's body is, I explain the desire for cremation. She examines the documents and assures us that there is no impediment to doing our bidding. I mention my son's desire to have a non-religious ceremony and she presents me with a list of 'Humanist' practitioners who will undertake to lead the service.

As in all things the matters lead to costs and choices, I am presented with a menu of types of caskets, cars, flowers, what should we dress the body in, what kind of shroud? I become impatient, I make decisions very quickly. There will be no viewings of my son's body, the body will not be dressed in any fancy clothes, expenditure will be sensible. I am sure, deliberate and precise. My boy would approve. I have a momentary thought that I should consult but I dismiss it quickly. We are done; we have agreed the cold business of money, made an appointment with a humanist practitioner who is nearby.

The young lady bids us farewell, and leaves me comforted that all these arrangements will be safe with her.

My wife maintains a light rein on the conversation; her humour is light and cheering, she urges me gently on, understanding what has to be done.

We find the home of the humanist practitioner; it is a few miles distant and set off the main road near a canal marina. It is a neat house set back off the road, with pretty grounds that are well looked after. We are greeted by a man a good deal younger than us, he is about fifty five, he is dressed in a suit, has a polished face, wears glasses; he is neat like the house.

We sit, awkwardly, at first but he soon makes us at ease and it is not long before I am opening my heart about my boy; his failings, his strengths, his history as I see it, my regrets, my failures, and in some depth about my boy's last days.

I understand that he must find out about my boy, his connections, his history , however at first I am not prepared, but the humanist minister, I could only think of the word minister though he insisted on a more secular title of Officiant, puts me at my ease. We talk for an hour; my wife from time to time gently intervening when I exaggerate, as she sees it, my guilt and my inevitable assertion that my boy went 'off the rails' because I left home when he was sixteen.

This repetitive refrain of my guilt irks her; she tells me that if every child from a fractured home 'went off the rails' the country would be awash with misfits.

Our humanist friend probes about my boy's relationships; his children, his former partner, and his friends; I am surprised by how much or how little I know about him outside his immediate family. I am slightly ashamed as I listen to my catalogue of contempt for those my boy held close. I hear myself and I am shocked.

It begins to dawn on me that this whole issue of a non christian ceremony will be very different from my entrenched view; I am gently cajoled into accepting the essential difference between religious and non religious ceremonies. I am persuaded that the music should be; not my choice, but the choice of his daughter, his sister, and reflect my boy's tastes. I shudder at the thought but smile at the same time. We discuss what I want to say, what I would like; I commit to writing a brief eulogy that I will aspire to read myself.

We have a date set for the cremation, we agree with the 'minister' a timetable for various actions and contacts, I give him all the details so that he can speak to all those I believe will be important in getting a fair picture of my boy. The minister promises to keep in touch and we will develop a form of ceremony that he believes will be appropriate for my boy. What is appropriate? I ask myself, I am filled with an anxiety that we must hit the mark; but how?

This is an unusually stressful meeting, although our m inister is extremely skilled at putting his 'clients' at their ease. Here is someone I have never met before and I am pouring out my soul within minutes of meeting him. My wife is by my side, listening and invigilating to ensure my expressions are sensible and my hysterical extremes of comment kept within reasonable limits. Not for first time, I am glad she is at my side.

The meeting comes to an end, we are bidden a warm farewell by the minister, I leave feeling relieved that we are in good hands.

My wife and I repair to a canal side restaurant that has just opened for the season. It is glum; we order a meal and drinks, which match the ambience of the establishment. I cannot but help remember that just over a week ago I was with my boy on this very canal albeit a few miles away, reflecting what life might be like living on a narrow boat. I do not weep, but smile ruefully and I share the experience for the first time with my wife; I find comfort in the memory. The next moments pass in silence. The canal is deserted, there is no ripple on the green water, the willows hang still, it is time, these things tell me, to be quiet, to gather myself, for what happens next will in large part be etched in my boy's memorial.

Grief persists, nagging away and tearing up my day after day. Where I live, the drama of my loss is impersonal, my neighbours and friends have been and are only vaguely aware of the sad events that have passed. They are also uncomfortable that my boy's passing was in the context of drug addiction. This makes them unsure. They bow their collective heads and shuffle by, avoiding the intimacy of sharing my grief. Apart from my wife, who is also a somewhat detached observer, there is no one close enough to share the pain. In the case of my wife she shares by default of her love for me, in my heart of hearts I have little idea of what she thinks of my boy, his life, his virtues or his demise.

"I Grieve."
I know you love me,
Yet you tip toe round my grief,
You are afraid
to touch the open wound.

I know you love me,
And I know you are afraid
To hold me,
 or just give me time to chat.

I know you love me
You don't know what to give
A smile, a minute
A hug, a greeting on the mat.

I know you love me
And all I want from you
Is just the time of day
To talk of this or that.

I know you love me
So come and share a prayer
Hold my hand and shed a tear
You know that's where I'm at.

I know that you love me
So please don't walk away
Grief is not a gift I bring
Just help me bear the pain.

The days pass, I am two people; one living apparently normally in one community, the other hiding away tortured by grief and regret. I am the same man, schizophrenic; living as if nothing untoward has happened whilst at the same time wracked with guilt for the loss of my boy.

At home I hide myself away and write; this is my refuge where I can speak to my darker spirits. I write:

 Now that you've gone?
My body and heart ache with your passing,

My mind is dominated by the memory of you,
your image, your wan face, your gentle smile.
I see the world as it is without you,
Much the same as it has always been.
Yet you're still there, aching for attention,
The idea of you, lingers, painful but full of smiles.
Grief; I can't avoid the term, lives on,
Though, with practice, it becomes my friend.
An uncomfortable friend to be sure
But you have gone away forever.

Why is grief so painful?
Is it because I'm so weak and perhaps regretful?
I don't know, except I regret you not being here with
me
I regret I did not love you more.
How sad is this, the more I love you,
The more I regret your passing.
'Passing' is not a true expression
For you stay rooted, insistent in my being.

CHAPTER SIXTEEN

I begin to write the eulogy for my boy's funeral, I am not sure if I write for him or for me, for my story is about us. I know this should not be, but it is all I can do since I have known him anew for these short ten weeks; his life before, another life and another person altogether. We have learned to know each other again, to love each other again. I have had a glimpse of his family and particularly of his children, and it is only a glimpse. I have managed to make a shallow connection with my eldest granddaughter, but I have hardly registered with the younger and not at all with his adopted son.

There are three epochs that define us, before I left home, the twenty five years of virtual estrangement and the last ten weeks.

I see his picture on my wall a chubby eighteen month year old, photographed in my arms some forty years ago, I remember the sweetness of his silky skin, his innocent bright eyes and his easy treacly chuckle, he was such an easy child to love. And love him we did, his mother and me. I remember him falling through the bannisters and crashing down the stairs, our terror at his injuries, the biggest black eye one ever saw.

His entrance a few months later to West Africa was spectacular, having kept a whole jet liner load of passengers awake all night, he swaggered into Kano in his striped shirt and blue shorts throwing the immigration and customs staff of that rough house airport into oohs! and aahs! What a lovely child. He was irresistible.

I remember how brave he was when I took him back to boarding school when he was not well, and he became progressively worse the further we travelled, but he did not once ask me to go back home, though I cannot believe he would possibly have not wanted to do so.

But worst of all I remember telling him and his sister, they were sixteen and fourteen respectively, that I was leaving home to live with someone else. I know I ripped the heart out of the family; it hurt the children as I knew it would. I had agonised about the pros and cons of my own fulfilment and the sacrifice of others, though I dare say that at the time I did not see it as I see it now. I cannot put aside the proposition that in that dreadful decision hung the future of my children's destiny. I had looked after my own happiness and sacrificed theirs. Have I been a thief who stole my boy's happiness? It is an indictment I find hard to bear.

Perhaps my worst sin was my denial of what I suspected and what my second wife understood; that my boy was on drugs. This was an appalling failure. There was and is no excuse, I stuck my head in the sand because I did not want to face up to the fact that my son has been a drug addict since his early twenties. I did little except make feeble enquiries, I never stood my ground because it meant standing up to his mother and making us do something, anything to help our boy from destroying himself. Now it is too late, to change things, to call back lost times. All that is left is to write a eulogy for a lost soul; my boy.

And so I write his eulogy:

I see the light that starts to fade,
I see the things that might have been.
I imagine the times together; father and son
like friends looking forward to the future.
I see too, a longing for the things that could have been,
and sadness for all the lonely days.
So soon, we have to part, so let us bury all the hurt

and be thankful that we are together.
The time we have is neither short, nor long, it is eternal.
So let me be thankful for the joy you bring
now that you've come home to me.
For home in my love, you will always stay
My son who was lost; but now is home again.

I write lines like the ones below but they are censored out by my wife who does not or refuses to believe my place in all this tragedy.

You went away, pushed out by selfish father,
Hid in dark places, looked the other way,
Abandoned in despair, rudderless through early
manhood
Finding hasty love, redeemed by children of your
own
Who love you still, and you have kept their faith
So good a father an example to the past
Lost and self destructed; each day the addiction has
its way
So down and down, lone soldier, looses lonely
battle
Parentless and lost, the end inevitable, the end – it's
here.

I continue to the approval of my censor, knowing that the lines are steeped in politeness, sentimentality and half truths. I am a hypocrite to the last, knowing full well that I am at best ambivalent about the grandchildren, who are still smoking, living in a culture I cannot even pretend to understand. I hope deep down that my older granddaughter will give me a sign that she cares, and after all we have been through, we will have a bond that may last. The hope is not convincing, the last three lines of my eulogy entreat the youngster

to at least take on the gentleness of their father, for
above all things, this was his strength.

Now that things are nearly done, it's time
to count the goodness of your days.
You brave little boy who followed snakes,
who charmed the people of that far off land
so blonde, so bright so full of life.
Our boy we sent away to school
So sweet, so gentle, and yet so innocent;
the madcap biker, who returned, as crazy as a coot,
A young dad embracing kids with love and
happiness
Some trials – sure! But lots of good times too.
But now your children can stand on better ground
three lovely kids, who'll make their journey,
and take your gentle kindness, to light their way -
through life.

CHAPTER SEVENTEEN

I continue to live my bifurcated life, one when I'm home and no one knows or knew my boy, or on the phone to the other world where grief and confusion rules each day.

My Boy's mother is still an enigma; we have not been able to talk about the real issues of why we let our boy go so far off the rails. We share compassion for his loss but we fail to face our responsibilities for failing our son. We blame each other but of course we don't come out and say it. She blames me for leaving her all those years ago, and I blame her for sitting by and watching our boy every day deteriorate into the emaciated wreck he became.

We, his mum and me, had talked about it directly only once or twice. The last occasion was about eighteen months before. I had over the years made an effort to meet him regularly.

I would meet my boy some place between our respective homes, usually in a pub where we would have a meal and a drink. He never drank very much, and ate sparingly in the latter years. Our relationship had been hard to sustain, he had become less and less communicative, it was always hard to have a meaningful conversation. Our meetings always took the same format. We would meet, we would hug, and then I would lead an interrogative conversation that almost always took the same form:

"How are you? How's your Mum? How's work? How's the kids?" His replies became almost entirely monosyllabic. The only consistent response outside "OK" was about work, he always said how tough it was, how he didn't earn enough, and how he struggled to make ends meet. For many years this tale of woe always resulted in me offering some cash to help. When that was done, I would then launch into a monologue about what was going on in my world. As soon as he could; he would bid me an urgent farewell, he'd take his money and run.

My second wife, now deceased, the one I left home for, observed year after year and eventually came out and said it: "He's on drugs." I heard her and I knew in my heart of hearts that she was probably right. Eventually she urged me to take my boy out, but not to consistently give him money. Use credit cards she would say, take no money, so you're not tempted to give away more money for... We never mentioned drugs again.

After a while as I enforced the ban on gift aiding, he'd not turn up at all; even if I'd driven the forty or fifty miles to our meeting place. In the last years I'd only met him twice, and on the last occasion in a ghastly pub he looked drawn and wan. After our sad meeting which was more monosyllabic than ever, I spoke to his mother who said, "You know our Boy, he's a law unto himself, he doesn't eat much and he's very solitary."

"Don't you think he's on drugs?" I asked, the line went quiet, "Oh no, perhaps he's smoked a little pot, but drugs, oh no, don't worry about that."

And so it was, I chose to turn my back on what was obvious, except perhaps to a parent who despite all, loves his son.

It occurs to me now that perhaps his mother knew, but was coerced into keeping the awful secret. It must have caused her untold pain, and I am sad she saw in me someone she was unable to trust. I suspect my boy coerced her into keeping the secret from me; through fear? I hope not. More likely from a fear of the regime that we might, as a team, have instigated. Even now it's hard to believe that the grip of addiction can overpower not only rational judgement, but love and care as well.

Today there is no more turning away; arrangements and spreading the news consume my time. I am mildly concerned about meeting the family of my former wife, I have not set eyes on them for so many years. How strange it will be, I wonder what they think of me and whether they share the view that my boy was destroyed by my fecklessness.

I spend a good deal of my time liaising with my daughter and the humanist gentleman preparing the order of ceremony/service for the funeral. I am all at sea, there is no familiarity about what is about to come to pass. No Vicar, no hymns, no blessing, even the chosen music is so alien to me I cannot help but shudder. The music is chosen between me, granddaughter and my daughter.

The week passes and the day of his funeral is here. I dress in the traditional attire; dark suit, white shirt black tie. My boy would scoff, I think and would prefer us all to turn up in jeans and tee shirt. Today's the day I must face the family of my first wife, it is some thirty years since I last met them all. We drive the familiar fifty miles to his mother's house; it is another bright summer morning. There are knots of people dotted about, some smoking in the garden, others clutching tea cups in tight groups in the little house. My wife is apprehensive she has never met my boy's mother before, we hold hands as we brave the throng.

Everyone is convivial, my former wife's family are all most pleasant, they pay their respects and offer their sympathy. My wife meets my former wife and they soon smile and seem to get on well. My daughter and her partner arrive and I feel a blessed sense of relief. We chat amiably and aimlessly waiting for the hearse. It arrives promptly at the appointed hour. We arrange the family group, so I travel with my former wife, my boy's children and my daughter. The air conditioning in the limousine does not work, I am aggravated, the grand children smell of tobacco; I am irritated but say nothing.

CHAPTER EIGHTEEN

We arrive at the crematorium; down the solemn leafy avenue just as the last party is leaving, the conveyor of cremations runs smoothly to time. There is a sizeable crowd around the entrance, I assume for the person in front of us. I am wrong. I see faces of old friends who have come to support me, friends of my daughter who I have seen fleetingly in the past, but the majority I do not know, perhaps one or two, but all the rest must be friends of my boy. There must be a hundred or more people, some dressed appropriately in jeans and tee shirts, some young ladies as if they were off to a cocktail party, and some lads straight from work.

We follow his coffin into the chapel, and we file into the front row, I am self conscious and aware of all the attendees watching us; my boy's nearest and dearest.

The music is alarming, at least for me, it's called November Rain by Guns and Roses. It's noisy and to me barely musical, still I smile to myself, he would enjoy my discomfort in a matey sort of way.

"We are here today," announces the officiant, "to mourn my boy's death and to celebrate his life."

I find it hard to celebrate.

The officiant continues through 'thoughts on life' that are fair enough and then he moves into a Tribute which is a romanticised précis of my boy's shambolic life, his misdemeanours, his adventures – small light hearted references to his brushes with the law, some tales I had never heard before – all portraying my boy as a sort of comic Robin Hood. He trivialised his wrong doing, making witty references to my boy avoiding sniffer dogs at airports. He makes no reference to the misery of drug addiction, the sadness of his parents' breakup, his dyslexia or the agony of his end.

The tribute ended with references to my boy's own family his kids, and their affection for one another. Then he calls on me to read my poem, I am unsure if I can do it. I stand before the assembled throng and do my best. I choke at the words "but now is home again." I recover and make it shakily to the end.

The officiant continues his tribute with anecdotes gleaned from my daughter, there are tales of the unexpected, some poignant some quite funny. It is good to know that as brother and sister they had been such good companions in their youth and teens, before the darkness of the drugs.

Then to my surprise, my boy's elder daughter stands and turn to us all, "I'd like to say that I know my dad was not perfect, but to me he was the best dad in the world, and will always be the best dad that's ever been." She speaks well, although her voice is shaking with emotion, she has guts and character. I weep, as do many others.

This part of the service ends with an Indian poet, not sure of the source – is it a Red Indian or an Indian from India? Sounds like an American Indian, the sort of thing you'd hear in a romantic Western. I see the point.

Let us remember the good times, the laughter not the tears, the loving not the anger, the courage not the pain. I must try.

J.S.Bach's Air on a G string is piped in; a time for contemplation.

Our service leader, ever mindful of the next party waiting to cremate a loved one who are approaching with metronomic precision, brings us to the closing words with yet another American Indian poem. The last two lines especially stay with me.

"Leave me in peace and I shall leave you in peace and while you live let your thoughts be with the living."

I hear my boy; his voice is clear, "Stop beating yourself up, dad."

The service leader reminds everyone that the collection will go to the hospice.

Then there is the most horrendous noise, it's "Black on Black" by AC/DC

The funeral is over.

The coffin is enclosed by the curtains, and his body is consumed by the flames.

Outside the chapel there is a relieved hubbub, it is over, and there is a palpable feeling of relief. Many of those who attended approach me to shake my hand to speak to the other members of the families. I search out my granddaughter and hug her and tell her how proud her father would have been. We hug, she smiles and says "Thank you, Grandpa."

Old friends have travelled from Scotland to Cornwall to be with us, it is very humbling and warming to feel their support. Many of them having journeyed hundreds of miles are unable to say anything, they just hug us, pat me warmly on my back. Some say 'it must be awful', some say 'time will heal', 'rah' 'rah' 'rah', they all mean well, they all love me, and I am grateful beyond measure.

In the best traditions of the British/English funeral everyone is asked back to a Pub where we can share a drink, some food and talk about my boy and maybe get to know each other. I am disappointed that some folk who have driven hundreds of miles must dash back, but most come back to the Pub.

It is a lovely day, and we all sit inside and out in the lovely garden chatting about this and that, I meet some of the friends of my boy who are an eclectic bunch. Many worked with him in the building industry and all said how reliable he was, how good he was at his job as a plasterer. Most of these individuals are clean, good folk, kind individuals with families. There are lots of tales of my boy having good times, but too many stories that trail off with..."well you know your boy."

The party segregates into its comfort zones; my son's work mates, his family, his mother's family, my relatives (few) and friends, and the others. The others are few, but you can see from the shaking young hands and their furtive gestures that they are druggies.

Some are smart, some are untidy but all have a regard for my boy and I want to embrace them all. I circulate as best I can, and I determine to talk to those few who I think are in the shadow of danger. They are to the man, polite and genuine, I make a plea ever so gently, "Turn back, if you can," I say, "turn back", I gently stroke them and turn away hoping but not believing there will be a change.

To those who are friends of mine I spend much of the time extolling the virtues of the hospice care that was given to my son. I repeat the message to everyone; I am boring them I am sure.

The guests begin to drift away, my wife's family remain, I make pleasant inconsequential conversation, I enquire about sons and daughters I can barely recall, and edge toward the door. I bid his mother farewell with a peck on the cheek and we escape my wife and me. Now it is over.

EPILOGUE

Of course it is not over. It is still today and a year has passed. My boy's family have reassembled for the 'Planting of his ashes' in the garden of remembrance. It was in yesterday, a poignant little group we made. My daughter, his sister has since returned to that place, I assume to 'remember' to be 'near him' on his birthday. I understand her, she cherishes his memory.

I have no need to travel to that garden, I remember him every day. I do not remember the failures; his and mine. I do remember above all his gentleness and his zany humour, his love for his children and our cherished days when we held each other on the sun bathed canal bank. When we were companions as father and son should be. These brief eternal hours are amongst the most beautiful of my life, and I am thankful for them.

My boy; his name is Steven and I love him still.

About the author:
Anthony James wrote this memoir following the death of his son, he says it was very cathartic for him. Anthony is in his early seventies and though retired he now writes full time and is working on his third novel. His earlier works, "Smiles in Africa" a novel is already published and he anticipates his second novel "The Poisoned Banquet" being published in 2012 . He also writes for magazines and publications mainly in the Caribbean where he winters with his wife Dawn. He has one surviving daughter Victoria who all can see is a much loved daughter.j

Lightning Source UK Ltd.
Milton Keynes UK
UKOW050710160512

192665UK00001B/2/P